TEA &
CHEMO

TEA & CHEMO

Fighting cancer, living life

Jackie Buxton

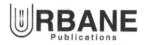

URBANE
Publications

urbanepublications.com

First published in Great Britain in 2015 by Urbane Publications Ltd
Suite 3, Brown Europe House, 33/34 Gleamingwood Drive, Chatham, Kent ME5 8RZ
Copyright © Jackie Buxton, 2015

A CIP catalogue record for this book is available from the British Library.

ISBN 978-1-910692-39-4
MOBI 978-1-910692-41-7
EPUB 978-1-910692-40-0

Design and Typeset by Julie Martin
Cover by Julie Martin
Printed and bound by CPI Group (UK) Ltd, Croydon, CR0 4YY

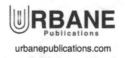

urbanepublications.com

In memory of **Julie**, **Ali** and **Mike**, and my YBCN friends,
taken so cruelly so young.

For **Lissie** and **Rosie**. I wish they hadn't had to have their mid-teens rubbed quite so violently in the rubbish of cancer, and I will never forget their faces when they learnt that I was ill. But they just got on with life, and didn't let a mum in and out of hospital with a memory eaten by Chemo Brain, or a dad distracted by looking after their mum, stand in the way of normality. I was proud of their spirit and relieved by their attitude. I hope they will look back and agree that it 'wasn't all bad'.

And for **John**. Because even when I was engulfed by the fear of waiting for the truth of my prognosis, when I was thick in the middle of treatments for cancer, I still felt like I was the luckiest girl alive to have him by my side.

Contents

1. Foreword

The warmth and love from friends and family, fellow writers, even friends of friends and complete strangers since my cancer diagnosis, has been quite overwhelming. I've blogged many times about how hard it is to feel too sorry for myself when people are enveloping me with love and kindness. Treatment for cancer is about keeping us alive and if people's loveliness is reminding us of just how wonderful it is to be alive, then how can we be upset or feel sorry for ourselves?

The fear of losing it all is stifling sometimes, but I could always remind myself that my treatment goal was cure. The true sadness of cancer is that this isn't the same for everyone. I have met several people younger than me who have developed secondaries and lost their lives – and at far too young an age. The tragedy of this takes my breath away. The thought of the partners, parents, friends and, not least, children, left behind is too awful to dwell on, and there isn't anything I can say to make that better.

To all those who aren't so lucky, to their family and friends, I dedicate this book.

WE ARE MACMILLAN.
CANCER SUPPORT

breast cancer now

1 Foreword

2. Why This Book ~ Tea & Chemo

When I was diagnosed with cancer I was swamped with factual information about the little blighter as well as the reasons for the treatments I was to have, together with their side effects. It was illuminating and helped me feel more secure. However there's a difference between knowing what's going to happen and knowing how it's going to feel.

As well as the facts, I wanted an honest account of the experience of cancer. What does it mean to lose your hair? I mean, *really mean*, emotionally? I wanted to hear it from someone who'd been there, done that and got the hat and wig and scarf to show for it. I wanted a book which would educate me in a softly, softly way. I wanted the author to be an ordinary person who was still enjoying life, who'd got through to the other side, and, crucially, done it without any Super Powers.

My aim is for **Tea & Chemo** to be that book. With my original blog posts as a framework and the addition of many more anecdotes, I hope that it will inform cancer sufferers and their loved ones whilst also making readers smile. All the blog posts were written as I tackled the disease. They are raw, real and honest and, I hope, give an insight into what it's like for anyone and everyone who is forced to cope with cancer, from diagnosis to treatment and beyond. It's information served with an empathetic and all-embracing hug, the story for around the camp fire or a cup of tea with friends on a lazy afternoon.

Since taking my first steps into the cavernous universe of cancer, I have learnt a little in my non-scientific, better-if-you-give-me-an-analogy kind of way about hormones (your body doesn't take kindly to you changing their levels), medicine induced water retention (who'd have thought to get rid of water retention, or 'Herceptin Bum', you should drink...err... water?), Vitamin D, Parabens, free make-up, eyebrow tattoos, Prosecco over white wine, Chemo Brain (it's for real and it sucks but it gets better), chemotherapy, radiotherapy, hormone therapy, tea therapy (ok, I made that one up) and time (that one's also true because time really does help you get used to – and deal with, anything).

Tea & Chemo is about sharing what I've learnt. It's here to hold your hand when chemo gives you a mouth full of ulcers, your bones feel like they've been squeezed in a vice and you just want to go to bed and wake up when the whole darned cancer thing has been sorted. I hope it will give you a hug when all your food tastes as though it's been sprinkled with bicarbonate of soda and stirred with mud. And I hope it will help your loved ones, too.

And I know some chemo secrets. I know that white sauce (sweet, not savoury) and rich tea biscuits are the only things which taste as they should in the first two weeks after a dose of chemo, and quite frankly, this is a time in your life when you can eat five bowls of white sauce on the trot (I did) and even mash a packet of biscuits guilt-free into the bowl.

You see, treatment has its perks.

3.
Fighting Cancer, Living Life:

The Blog Posts

Pebbles: the beginning

Sometimes a pebble is thrown onto the path we're walking and we trip before staggering slowly back to our feet. Every time a sizeable pebble has been thrown in my direction I've sought solace in writing, either in my own in the form of a diary, or in that of others – which has been tricky. Whenever I've wanted to find real life stories of people who've faced similar pebbles and, most crucially, are walking upright again, I haven't really found them.

When my boyfriend died when he was only 17, I searched for that book but I never found it. Years later I vowed I'd write a version of my story in the hope it might comfort people in their darkest moments that there IS life after the death of a loved one, even at 16 when the world is still so gloriously black and white. But I never wrote it.

When my daughter had a stroke, at only 15 small months of age, I devoured websites, support groups, non-fiction and even fiction to find an inspirational story of a baby with half her body paralysed who'd gone on to lead a happy, fulfilled life. And even though I know the world is packed with such success stories now, my 13 year old daughter being one of them, I couldn't find the story I craved back then.

So, now I learn that I have breast cancer and the path of the next few months – and years – will be littered with pebbles en-route to what I pray is a full recovery.

But this time, I've decided that I am going to write it down.

I'm going to blog about the journey. But I want my posts to have purpose, not just to be cathartic for me, but with the aim of calming a few nerves for those in a similar position who are perhaps a little further back on the road. So I will only post when I feel I have something positive to say, something I've felt or learnt which might help someone in a similar position. It won't be for everyone – already I fear my humour is lurching a little into the macabre – but if I can pass on the message that having cancer is not all bad, then I'll call that a success.

You know, it's really hard to feel down when so many people are showering you with love and caring. Love really is what makes the world go round; or should be anyway.

The not knowing

At diagnosis, the most terrifying aspect of it all was the *not knowing*. Has it spread? I asked. We don't know, they said. It's aggressive – heart sink. It's fast growing – sinks further. Grade three – ends up in toes. We think we've caught it early. But by this time I wasn't really listening.

And with the *not knowing* comes *the wait*. It's the well-documented fear of the unknown, and a time when the brain doesn't just do the roller coaster but has a spin on the waltzer as well. There's the wait for the mastectomy, the operation you crave to cut away this cancer from your body to stop it building further cancer cells, to put you a step further along the path to the place you were in before you had cancer. You're told that the two or three week wait will have no effect on prognosis. You know it's right. The medical profession have to tell you the truth because otherwise you'll sue. That's just how it is these days. And if you take the heart out of this equation, it's cheaper for the NHS to treat cancer in the earlier stages so if a few days made a difference to the extent of treatment needed, you can bet your bottom penny that the NHS would find a way to carry out the operation earlier. That's what I told myself, anyway.

But it didn't change anything. I still wanted that operation *today*. I didn't even want to go home, would have preferred to have been whisked off to a hospital bed and woken up with a dressing to mark the spot where the cancer had been, rather than waking up to the haunting realisation that I had cancer. And if I needed any reminding, well there it was: neatly packaged in a lump for me to prod and examine and decide that yes, definitely, it had grown in the past few hours.

It's an odd concept that you're whiling away the days before a part of you that is so bound up in who you are, is going to be cut away. I guess you just want to feel like you're doing something positive to take a step closer to life as it was before you had to deal with the *not knowing* and *the wait*.

It's a strange place you enter when you cross through that door marked cancer.

I was given the choice of mastectomy before chemo or chemo followed by mastectomy. The prognosis was identical, apparently.

Is there not even a single 0.00001% of a degree in it, I asked.

Not one, I was told.

The principle is that if you cut away the source of the cancer with a mastectomy, there is no engine room left to create new cancer cells. And you're not just closing down the engine you're digging it out and consigning it to the scrapheap. What's more, before incineration, it will be subjected to a thorough examination to tell you exactly what type of engine it was. It doesn't stop there because the foundations and supporting walls around the engine will be demolished too. This made perfect sense to me. I liked the idea that the surgeons would take away more than the engine and that I would get my definitive pathology report as to exactly what we were dealing with. I'd have my *not knowing*, answered.

But there is another way of looking at it. There may – who knows? It's that pesky *not knowing* again – be some stray cells paddling around in our circulatory systems. Starting with chemo would hopefully eradicate such stray cells and reduce the size of the tumour for good measure. Sometimes this can reduce the need for a mastectomy to a lumpectomy where most of the breast is saved. Although a lumpectomy was never an option for me.

It's hard to believe that there isn't an advantage in one system over another. But there isn't and so it becomes a matter of personal choice.

I chose the operation before chemo because I didn't want to see or feel the lump any longer than I needed to. And I also wanted the information the pathology report on the removed tumour would provide. In the case of chemo first, such information is gleaned via scanning and that wasn't clear-cut enough for me.

It was the right choice for me. It meant I got the good news that my actual tumour was smaller than the diagnostic ultrasound had suggested. It had reduced from 2.5cm to 1.9cm (although the surrounding 'pre-cancerous' area – where cells have developed abnormalities but the abnormalities have not yet (nor may ever) spread to other breast cells – remained the same at 5cm). The accurate measurement of the grade 3 tumour dipping below 2cm put me at a slightly earlier stage of cancer which was the best news I'd had since that first fateful diagnosis.

Unfortunately the operation also revealed that one of my lymph nodes was cancerous and thus I had to have a further operation to remove all of those. Three of these showed cancer so again, in my circumstances, with news not as good as I'd dared to hope, it calmed me to think that the engine house had gone.

It's slightly unnerving when O-level Biology was the bane of your school life, to be faced with these scientifically-driven decisions about your future. However, I have been reminded on several occasions that I wouldn't be asked to make a decision on anything for which the medical profession had a clear view on the right course. For example, the grade and size of my tumour, together with my age, meant that the decision to have chemo was never in question. On diagnosis I was told I would have a mastectomy and chemo and that, emphatically, was that. Of course you have the right to refuse treatment but the consequences would be expressly explained to you and this would be an exercise in your human rights, not in medical choice.

And so, two weeks after my mastectomy operation, I met with the surgeon who went through the pathology report. Hearing the cancer was in my lymph nodes was very unsettling. My oncologist tried to explain logically how the medical profession still felt confident that the cancer was unlikely to have spread further than the breast and lymph nodes, without putting me through a whole body scan. I was quite jumpy about this. I thought I'd have preferred the opportunity for the peace of mind of a scan – and, again, an end to the *not knowing*. However, I've heard that scans can have the opposite effect of creating calm. We all have spots and blemishes on the inside as well as the outside, apparently, and the scan picks them all up. The patient is alerted to every smudge in their system, which is most unlikely to be cancer but must, nonetheless, be vigorously monitored. The stress of that can be overwhelming.

I was told that three out of my 18 lymph nodes were affected and that staff didn't routinely scan until four or more had signs of cancer. This knowledge was meant as a comfort. It wasn't. I was only one lymph node away from needing a scan. I 'almost' wished I'd had four lymph nodes affected, at least then I'd have a scan, at least then I'd 'know'.

I wanted a scan but I didn't want to need one. The waltzer ride was ramped up again and the attendant had given my chair an extra spin.

The oncologist said one thing which went the furthest to putting my fears at ease. He said that he wasn't a fan of scanning and that even in patients where most of their lymph nodes were affected, that's say, 15 out of 18 (or 22 or 16 – there is no set amount of lymph nodes), many of those patients would still prove to be completely clear of cancer in the rest of their body. The lymph nodes were doing their job, containing the cancer from progressing further and in many cases, successfully.

All his studying at med school and his experience thereafter was worth it for me right there, in that single answer. I haven't given the lymph nodes too much thought since that day and

I certainly don't wake up in a panic anymore. Remember, even if you are faced with a higher proportion of lymph nodes affected, my oncologist would say that there's still a good chance the cancer was stopped right there.

I wasn't keen to have another operation to remove the lymph nodes. I really wanted to crack on with chemo. It would take 18 weeks to complete my six courses but I couldn't begin counting down until I'd started. I just had to tell myself that the lymph node removal was another one of those steps in the positive direction of being Cancer Free. My father-in-law leaned into me a few days after my original diagnosis and simply whispered, A to B, B to C, C to D. And that was it. In those few words he told me that I had to look at the smaller steps en-route to cancer obliteration, rather than tackling the overwhelming task of everything all at once. I suppose it's simply another way of saying, 'Take one step at a time!' but somehow, this was much more powerful. I repeated the mantra throughout treatment and it really worked for me. With the lymph node removal, we were now at stage C in proceedings.

Two weeks after the lymph node removal, or axillary clearance, I finally started chemo.

I liked having chemo. Or put it another way, I enjoyed the process and the confidence it gave me that my body and the medical profession combined were too powerful for any delinquent cells. We'd grabbed this cancer by the horns, torn it to shreds in the operating theatre, and now I had the most powerful of vacuum cleaners to absolutely sanitise the area so that we could all wash our hands of the little blighter.

I remember going into hospital with my husband for my first session of chemo and feeling a great surge of relief. The waltzer slowed down, spinning relatively peacefully to a controlled, manageable cadence which I could cope with. From this point forward, we were solely employed in evacuation and bolting the door against any return. The waiting for results regarding this cancer was over. And that was a wonderfully liberating feeling. I felt that in the Jackie Buxton versus Cancer match, I'd gained some semblance of control.

Now, a year after my final chemo in June 2014, I can categorically state that of all the operations and treatments, and even including the taking of the tiresome Tamoxifen (better known as Tamoxibollox), that the time of *not knowing* was positively the worst of it all.

If you're at this stage, hang on in there. Honestly, it gets easier.

Blood, Blood, Glorious Blood

I'm going to talk about blood – not the messy, congealed kind but the type stashed away neatly in hospital blood banks. Before I get going, I should explain that what happened to me was an extremely rare side-effect of the surgery to remove my tumour and not to be feared if you have to undergo the same procedure. Indeed, even when it does occur, the results are not always so dramatic – but then I'm a writer and I'll do anything for a good story.

Following my initial surgery I suffered a rather dramatic spurting artery and lost lots of blood. After two transfusions and the injection of so much saline fluid I looked like a puffer fish (followed by three more pints of blood in the emergency surgery which followed), I emerged happy to be here and oh so grateful that people of my blood group happened to give blood recently.

I'd been giving blood regularly thanks to a poignant donor campaign when I was a student. Every four months I'd pop along to my local mobile centre, chat with the nurses, eat all their biscuits and toddle along home feeling very virtuous. For anyone who hasn't given blood or received it before, I should say that a large chunk of the 30-45 minute process is taken up with screening to limit the risk of disease spreading through your blood to a patient, and the blood is rigorously checked for infection after you've given it.

When I woke up alive and well and more than a little proud of the bruise from shoulder to hip, and the marvelling from staff at just how much blood had been squeezed into one so small, I was relieved that I'd given blood in the past. Who'd have thought that one day it would be who me who needed it?

I knew that I wouldn't be allowed to give blood anymore* and consoled myself with the fact that at least I'd given blood for the past twenty years. And then I worked it out. Four monthly giving is the maximum allowed for women (three monthly for men) so that the donor has ample time in between to build their blood supplies back up to normal levels. So it would have taken one person twenty months of giving just to provide the amount I needed to be sitting up again. On that basis, the potential amount of people I could have helped over my entire adulthood was a paltry twelve. Twelve! I was shocked.

Now, I know not everybody is going to need five pints, but nonetheless how much blood would we need in the banks if we had a natural disaster or an epidemic? Could there ever be a situation where I could have been lying there with the staff whispering, 'Hang on in there Mrs Buxton, we're just waiting for your blood to arrive from Newcastle, Edinburgh, John o' Groats…'?

There is a bright side to having cancer and that is that everyone wants to help. It's the loveliness of the human spirit; everyone wants to make it right and if they can't do that, they want to make it easier for you or more comfortable. Is this a good place to thank everyone for the cards, messages, flowers, chocolates, candles, moisturiser, fluffy socks and fleecy cardigans, touching charms and pieces of jewellery, books, DVDs, writing retreats (oh yes), magazines, cleaning, ironing, notebooks (you know how much I love my notebooks), offers of shopping, lifts, meals for my children, cake, bags of healthy cancer-fighting eating and meals-on-wheels on my doorstep and hugs and positive vibes? You're all sent from God.

But back to blood. I've realised that there is another way that people can directly help and it is this. If you can, please would you give blood? I've discovered only 4% of the population do. And please, tell your friends and family. You'll be helping me because I'm not allowed to give blood anymore and you'll be helping to save lives. I'm evidence of that. It's that simple. Head to **http://www.blood.co.uk/information-for-patients/** to find out more and your closest place to give.

Let's get those stocks back up, I feel I've had more than my fair share of late. And to all of you who do regularly give blood, thank you from all of us.

Will a thumb print do?

It's a funny old world we live in. I'm so poorly that my husband's been called back into hospital in the middle of the night. I'm whispering messages to the nurse for my children, just in case. I need blood to save my life and have already signed the mastectomy consent papers to say that I would (yes please) accept a blood transfusion should the medical staff deem it necessary. The poor doctor, however, who just wants to get the blood administered, has to wait until he's read me the comprehensive list of potential side-effects associated with giving me the blood, so that I won't sue the NHS in the future. Ironically, if I hadn't signed for the blood, I wouldn't have been around to sue the NHS anyway. Not that I was particularly aware of what I was signing – I was so poorly, I could barely make sense of what he was saying. I'd love to have seen my signature that day. I wonder if they let me do a thumb print?

Now, I'm not belittling the risks of having someone else's blood in my body. Having five pints of somebody else's blood squeezed into me wasn't on my bucket list. But when the side effect of not taking the blood is death, I think there should be a way of saying, just give it to me now, goddamnit.

After the operations

Most mastectomy operations happen perfectly smoothly. You'll wake with the wound hidden behind a tight dressing and will be sporting an attractive 'bag' or two called a 'drain', which is designed to collect excess fluid. This will be removed a few days later amidst much euphoria. Until then, I packed mine into a small bag over my shoulder which of course, had to go everywhere with me. A week later a male friend asked me why I wasn't putting my bag down – admittedly it was slightly odd to be sitting at the dinner table with a leather bag across my chest – and I said I needed it for my blood. Of course he then insisted on having a look. I'm constantly amused by the Venus and Mars of men and women. My female friends never asked, it never occurred to me to show them and my daughters positively recoiled at the sight of it.

As with all operations, your mastectomy is a great opportunity to hog the sofa. There's absolutely no lifting allowed in the first few days following the operation and boy, that kettle can be heavy, best to let everyone else make you a cuppa for the first week, ok? In fact I think it's enshrined in medical law.

Your movement is very limited in the first few days after the operation. I remember being given a leaflet in advance which showed exercises for the arm during the first week post-mastectomy, and scoffing. As if I wouldn't be able to roll my shoulder backwards and forwards or raise my hand to shoulder height!

I couldn't.

But once I'd got the first movements back, the rest followed quickly. I won't tell you how soon I went running after the operation as I will be in trouble with the nurses, but I will admit that it was sooner than recommended. I'm not condoning this reckless attitude but hope it serves to show that normal movement can be resumed very quickly. I would advise that you do your exercises whenever you can, however. I would do mine morning and night and again every time I boiled the kettle. That way I wouldn't forget. I did them frequently but never forced them past the point stated by the physios. Honest (actually, that bit is true).

Cording

I had quite severe cording from my armpit down to beyond my elbow after my operations. I suspect my body didn't take too kindly to having three operations in quick succession. Cording, or Axillary Web Syndrome (AWS), is scar tissue in the arm and is a fairly common side-effect of surgery. Mine looked like a sinewy tree branch, running quite prominently along the underside of the arm, but I've read that it can present as a clump of smaller branches, more like roots. So prominent was my 'branch', I could have got a good grip on it with the other hand, had I felt so inclined.

Cording isn't painful but it needs to be rectified or you'll struggle stretching your arm to its full extent again. If you're going to have radiotherapy, it needs to be sorted fairly swiftly so that you can raise your arm above your head while the treatment takes place.

Your Breast Cancer Nurse (BCN) or a lymphoedema physio will give you exercises to stretch the affected area until it's loosened off – or rather, until the scar tissue has snapped. This is a much more pleasant experience than it sounds. I actually heard my cording 'pop' on a few occasions. It was the sound of the scar tissue breaking down and with it came much more movement. I became quite obsessive about how far I would dare to push my exercises in search of the 'pop'. I was told by the physio that there was no harm in pushing it; in fact she encouraged her clients to push it as far as they could bear.

It reminded me of when I stuck my arm in a spin drier which, unfortunately, was still spinning. I know, I know. Brilliant surgeons stitched me back together again and a wonderful physio put me through my paces to afford me as much movement as possible in an arm and wrist which had been broken too many times to count. Without the use of my left arm, I quickly learnt why you need two – for essential tasks such as carrying a sandwich AND a drink at the same time, to opening post and eating peas with a fork.

Taking off my make-up at night was another problem, as pouring lotion onto a cotton wool ball is a two-handed procedure. I was forced to use make-up remover wipes which gave me spots. I was not happy. I was debilitated and had a face full of spots at the age of 32 when quite frankly, I felt I was a little too old for them.

After a couple of weeks of physio I could incline my forearm to around 45 degrees of a bicep curl, which, although progress, wasn't of great use to anyone. The physio had told me to go further. She said that scar tissue could be as hard as bone but that I had to break it down. One night, increasingly annoyed at the sight of my spotty face in the mirror, I decided I was going to squeeze the most offensive blemish. But it's very difficult with one hand when you can't get a grip. It was the perfect moment to give the bicep curl its 'push'.

I stood in front of the mirror, my eyes streaming with the pain, my fist inching closer to my shoulder but still miles away from my face. And then it happened. Just like that. With one final push it popped, my fist punching my face as the blockage released. The scar tissue was gone, I could flex my arm in and out like the old days, and never, ever, has squeezing a spot been quite so pleasurable.

I decided to do something similar with my cording but in a less extreme way as, post-mastectomy and lymph node clearance, we all have to be careful of the risk of lymphoedema. It worked. I still have a slight train track effect under my arm but more importantly, have no restriction in movement. Whilst I can't claim to be doing my exercises quite as meticulously as before, I do practice them most.

Fighting Cancer, Living Life

Post-surgery arms are prone to stiffening up and these exercises also help keep lymphoedema at bay.

Lymphoedema

The lymphatic system is the body's clean-up team. It sends extra fluid to stressed areas of the body to clear out dead cells and toxins and fight infection. Primarily Axillary Clearance, or the removal of lymph nodes, but also radiotherapy, chemo and other cancer treatments, as well as the cancer itself, can damage the lymph system so that it struggles to remove the excess lymph fluid once its work is done. This can result in lymphoedema, a pooling of the lymph fluid in the body.

I was first told of the risk of lymphoedema on that fateful day I learned I had cancer. During the mastectomy operation, the surgeon would also remove the 'sentinel node(s)', the first node, or nodes in the path to take lymph fluid away from the breast. If the sentinel node proved to be clear of cancer, no further surgery would be required. However, an Axillary Clearance would be unavoidable if cancer was found in the sentinel nodes. This was considered to be best practice to put as few people at risk of lymphoedema as possible.

Isn't lymphoedema just a fat arm? I asked. In the world of bizarre decisions into which I'd been unceremoniously plunged, I'd have chosen a fat arm over the threat of further surgery at a later date. The surgeon and Breast Cancer

Nurse both smiled (I've realised since writing about my first meeting with the surgeon and BCN that whilst I was not at my sunniest, they did a lot of smiling) and said that it was a little more complicated than that. A fluid filled arm was an incapacitated, heavy arm which struggled with basic tasks and was open to infection. It was something to be avoided if at all possible.

Once I'd found out that my sentinel node was affected, I just wanted all those lymph nodes out. A fat, incapacitated, heavy arm which struggled with basic tasks was of no concern to me then. That said, after the previous joys of artery spurting, I approached the operation with much more foreboding than usual.

What if my arteries were prone to be the inappropriately bleeding kind?

In the past I'd never been particularly nervous of operations. I'd had enough to know that my body could cope with a general anaesthetic and quite enjoyed the experience of being told to do nothing. And there's something very gratifying about that first cup of tea, and toast if you're lucky, after the obligatory starving before the op. The starving is certainly the worst part of it for me. What, not even a measly cup of tea? Artery spurt notwithstanding, in the past I'd woken up in a much better state than when I'd gone in.

This time it was different. I knew in my rational moments that it was extremely unlikely that an artery would bleed again. The surgeon was not going to let it happen twice. But my biggest fear for the Axillary Clearance was that being pushed into the anaesthetist's room in that same hospital, on that same bed, with the same instructions and same routine, would give me a sort of out of body experience, a physical reaction, a panic attack. Off would spurt that damn artery again. I'd be dying on the table. But where in the past my brain would have jumped in saying, 'She is not dying here, mate, she's got way too many jobs to do,' and fought to get me out of the situation, this time I was worried a panic attack would play tricks on my brain and I'd lose my ability to fight.

Ridiculous, I know.

It's particularly ridiculous as I'd already had the emergency operation post artery bleed, and all had been well. However, I was mindful that before that particular operation, the pain had been a '10' on the 1 to 10 scale. I just needed the staff to do something – anything – to take the pain away; not to mention curtail the threat of bleeding to death.

Back to the Axillary clearance. It was absolutely fine. The silver lining was that while he was in there, the surgeon had the opportunity to clear up some of the detritus from the bleeding artery and subsequent emergency op, so that when I came out of this third operation, my arm felt much less sore than when I'd gone in. Having the lymph node operation go smoothly was good for me. It drew a line under the emergency. I no longer wonder if my arteries are the spurting type. They just got a bit excited on that particular occasion.

After three operations and recovery spanning six weeks, I couldn't help wondering whether it might be better to take out all the lymph nodes during the mastectomy operation. But now that I understand the lymphoedema risk and its side-effects, I do believe it is the right decision to test the lymph nodes before removal, even though it can necessitate a second operation later.

The threat of lymphoedema never goes away. The trick is to not tax your arm too much, particularly in a static position, which forces the body into 'protect mode'. This encourages the release of extra lymph fluid and is when a damaged lymph system is most at risk of lymph pooling.

It takes a little adjustment. A the beginning I used to forget that I wasn't meant to hold heavy shopping bags in my weak arm but now my brain has adjusted and doesn't even suggest I carry anything remotely too heavy. I would recommend finding a solution so that you avoid carrying too much in your good hand or worse, in the crook of your elbow. I did this and now have a stubborn incidence of tennis elbow in my 'good' arm which is nowhere near as much fun as it sounds and is incredibly hard to get rid of. And don't start me on the potential for hip and pelvis problems if you start loading

Fighting Cancer, Living Life

yourself up like a pack horse. I've bought a couple of bags, this lymphoedema risk has its perks, to try to distribute the weight over my back now that I'm one arm short. I'd recommend a rucksack – they don't all look like you're lost your way to Snowdon – and bags with long straps you can wear diagonally across your chest are also useful.

Lymphoedema isn't an excuse for a sedentary lifestyle, however. Weight increase is a risk factor in lymphoedema itself and non-stressful movement and exercise actually increase the efficacy of the flow of lymphatic fluid around the body, with contracting muscles helping to propel the lymph fluid through the lymph vessels. The key is to build up slowly to more strenuous exercise so that you put minimal stress on the body. And if you have time out, there's no going straight back to one armed planks; you have to start again and build up slowly.

*Incidentally, I've also had to take myself off the Anthony Nolan Trust donor (stem cells) list which helps people with blood cancers such as leukaemia. Would you take my place on the list? Head to **http://www. anthonynolan.org/8-ways** to find out more.

A Cold Cap

I'm not scared of spiders, nor would I jump on a chair if I saw a mouse. In truth I have few phobias, save for birds trapped in kitchens, but I blame that on the cat – RIP Gismo. Not that I ever witnessed the squalls and spitting feathers for more than a few seconds, you understand, before slamming the door behind me and yelling to my beleaguered mother to come and remove the irate bird from the scene.

But a demented bird is about it as far as phobias go. With one exception. The cold. Cold fingers and toes have driven me to tears on several occasions. I'd like to say that I have Raynaud's Disease but I can't actually claim it to be proven. Although I do know that however many pairs of gloves I wear when I walk, however many layers of Woollie Boolie socks and shoe covers I wear when I cycle, my extremities are always colder and whiter than everyone else's.

This fear of the cold invades my rational thought, sending messages to my brain when my ankles are lapped with cold water that this is a *dangerous situation*, that I should *evacuate immediately*, when the rest of my family and friends are bathing merrily, seemingly oblivious to the potential for the hideous effects of cold-induced brain freeze which threatens us all.

So why am I talking about the cold?

It's no secret that most people who undergo chemotherapy
for breast cancer lose at least some of their hair. I have
long hair and confess that the thought of being bald
distresses me slightly less than the prospect of finding large
clumps of matted, curly hair all over the carpet, in my
hands after combing, in the sink and, horror of horrors, on
my pillow.

Even the most beautiful of wigs can't prevent the hair loss on
the pillow.

When you're diagnosed with cancer, it's terrifying. However,
several actions quickly kick into play which help make it more
bearable. One of these is the allocation of a key worker, a nurse
specially trained in cancer care assigned to be your first point
of contact throughout treatment. When I realised that the
nurse who'd helped to break the news to me and my husband
was going to be with us every step of this bumpy cancer ride,
I could have jumped up and hugged her. She was so calm, so
comforting, and so knowledgeable, that I started to feel that
we'd be alright after all.

My key worker mentioned the Cold Cap. It's a tool which
may – 'may' being the operative word – prevent hair loss as a
result of chemotherapy. The process involves freezing the hair
follicles while chemotherapy is administered. The patient often
sits in warm blankets and gloves and is advised to take pain

killers before the cap is applied but nonetheless, the process isn't for the faint-hearted.

Did I mention I don't like the cold, my pathological fear of *ice cream head*?

When I heard the invention described as a 'cap' I imagined it to be a peaked affair with 'New Yorkers' on the front and ice pads pushed discreetly under the rim. Oh no. The cap in our Cold Cap would appear to be more like a thick, tight-fitting swimming cap, capable of administering temperatures of minus 30 degrees to the hair follicles all around the head.

So, I ask my nurse, what does it actually feel like to wear a Cold Cap?

Well, she says, I've heard that it's like the worst tooth ache but in your head.

OK.

But that only lasts for the first 15 to 20 minutes, after that the head just feels numb.

OK. That doesn't sound too pleasant either.

The other down side to the Cold Cap is that it has to be worn either side of treatment so that the hair follicles are frozen for the entire time the drugs are travelling around the blood. A typical one hour course of chemotherapy can thus take three to four hours. Do I really want each session to last the morning when I could be in and out of hospital and getting on with my day? You also can't hear and thus talk to others while you're wearing the Cold Cap which is something which doesn't come very easily to me.

But perhaps a little time and a lot of discomfort is worth it for the chance to keep your hair, to keep your sanity, to stop yourself ageing twenty years overnight and to prevent the ghastly clumps of hair on the pillow?

Perhaps. I change my mind daily.

I looked at the stats. Does it really work? I've scoured Mr Google and respected cancer charity forums and find success rates ranging from 20% to 75% with the odd site claiming even higher success rates based on the type of chemotherapy used. It's undisputed that the Cold Cap has some success in preventing hair loss entirely and, more commonly, in decreasing the amount of hair which goes. Unfortunately research doesn't tell us which hair the Cold Cap chooses to save. The advice is to have a wig in reserve and the National Health is kind enough to contribute to that.

And so I went wig shopping with my children last week. I had hoped we'd spend a few hours trying out outrageous wigs on each other, my teenage fashion aficionados stating categorically which wigs I could and couldn't carry off. Unfortunately it was a little more sombre than that and they were only allowed to advise. That said, we were unanimous on the decision and I'm excited about the potential new me which emerged from the appointment. But no clues as to the style of wig – even my hubbie hasn't seen it yet.

So, after musing over it for weeks, researching the hard facts and attempting to brush phobias aside, will I be using the Cold Cap?

Absolutely not.

But you might want to ask me again tomorrow.

Unashamedly spineless

I had my first dose of chemo this week. It was pretty much as expected. The staff couldn't do enough for me, the cups of tea were plentiful and we were even brought sandwiches and cake thanks to my session being fortuitously allocated to lunch time. After a saline drip was set up, the chemo was administered, in my case, through a cannula in the hand.

And that's it really. The rest of the time you sit and chat and wonder if you have enough eggs at home for Pancake Day – which we did although I wish I hadn't burnt the 'non-stick' pan a few weeks earlier.

I can't pretend it was a walk in the park. It generally feels as if I've had a murky pair of swimming goggles prised over my head resulting in smeared, wobbly vision, a crushing headache and morning sickness without the baby. Oh, and water tastes like flat Alka Seltzer stirred with a dash of mould. But it's one down and that means five to go which is better than where I was last week. And I'm another week closer to my ultimate goal of cancer in the past tense.

So, instead of pondering on the well-documented side-effects of chemo, I thought I'd let you know my decision.

Did I go cold?

When I write blog posts I hope that they might entertain and even provide a nugget of information but I don't really expect them to help me make life affecting decisions. However, the flurry of responses which came via Facebook and in person – thank you so much to everyone – really helped my thought process. I quickly realised that what I wanted to find was an excuse *not* to wear the Cold Cap; something we'd call in our house, 'an excuse to be a wuss', for fear it was spineless not to at least attempt to try it. Then a friend mentioned two of her friends who did use the Cold Cap. Unfortunately it had no effect for the first but in the case of the second it worked – ish – with her hair thinning but not falling out altogether. However, due to the thinning the friend hated her hair, primarily because of the special shampoos needed to minimise the hair loss, and the lack of serum, gel or mousse, hair-drying and curling or straightening. No products? I broached. What, no frizz-calming, curl taming products? I'd look like Tina Turner, I exclaimed, perfect in Mad Max 3, granted, but not, perhaps, in my village. And thinned, curly long hair? Roll over Rab C Nesbitt.

Crucially, the friend was glad she endured the ordeal because she was happy to have her own hair at the end of the treatment.

But, personally, I didn't go for the Cold Cap.

Instead I had my hair cut to ease the pain of it falling out. I picked up my wig from the wig shop. And I sat and thought about ice cream in pancakes rather than *ice cream head*.

And I'd made the right decision for me. Unashamedly spineless.

More about the cold cap

I think we will look back in the not very distant future and see the cold cap a little like we view Victorian swimming costumes today: functional, moderately effective but fairly excessive and positively no fun at all. For the moment, however, the head squeezing ice box is the best on offer. And it works for some people. If I were in charge of its evolution however, my priority would be to work out a way of knowing whose hair would and whose wouldn't respond favourably to it.

Am I pleased I didn't try it? Yes. Because for me, the chemo-receiving itself was the best part of the chemo cycle. It was the side-effects I wasn't so keen on. I know some people who wished they hadn't bothered: their hair fell out anyway. But I know others who are delighted they persevered. Even for those whose hair thinned, the growing back process was much easier. So, I'm afraid, until someone invents the, 'Whose hair works?' test, I can only really suggest you do what suits you.

Since my original blog post I've learnt that the big freeze doesn't stop at the hair follicles, there are ice mitts and ice slippers you can wear in an attempt to hold onto your finger and toe nails too. If this has a good chance of working, and you feel you might be able to bear the cold (you know my feelings on this) then I would be tempted to try them. Eight months after chemo (although perhaps exacerbated by Herceptin), I am still plagued by flaky nails which break off so far down the nail bed that I have little sores over the ends of my fingers. They are much more painful than they look and should elicit far more sympathy from others than they actually do!

So how was chemo?

I couldn't wait for chemo to start. I wanted the heavy duty cleaning mob to move in to my body and exorcise any so much as a suggestion of the disease. The sooner they cracked on with the job in hand, the sooner it would be finished.
Of course, I still had some trepidation about how my body would deal with chemo. It would be hard to sit through your four page briefing with the consultant, signing to say you understand everything, when really you've spent most of the time trying to keep your mind in the room and the reality that yes, this is really you sitting in this chair discussing chemotherapy - and not have some trepidation. However, what you don't learn in your pre-chemo consultation is how pleasant your chemo visits
will be.

No, really.

I began a programme of visiting the Sir Robert Ogden Macmillan Centre at Harrogate Hospital every three weeks for over a year of chemo followed by Herceptin infusions. The staff and volunteers treated me like a local celeb. Not that I'm special. They just made it their business to remember my name, everybody's name, and to find out a little about who we really are away from all this cancer nonsense. They bring sandwiches and cake. And blankets, because chemo can be cold as it's stored in the fridge. It's a very weird sensation when you feel a rush of cold fluid travelling through a vein in your arm. After the first session, I took plenty of layers with me.

And tea. They bring you magic pots of tea.

Before each chemo treatment, you're asked to fill out a detailed questionnaire about your tolerance to the side-effects you've experienced over the past three weeks since your previous infusion. Everybody reacts differently to chemo but you'd be unusual not to suffer any side-effects at all. However, those clever nurses will do their utmost to find a way to lessen the side-effects and they take your responses to the questionnaire very seriously.

There are different types of chemo for different cancers, and different types of chemo for different types of breast cancer. For my hormone and protein receptive cancer, I was given three sessions of Epirubicin (Pharmorubicin) followed by three lots of Docetaxel (Taxotere) over an eighteen week period. Different chemos have different side-effects and different people react to the different types of chemo differently.

For the first three sessions I felt a bit of a fraud. People were giving me so much sympathy, leaving meals on my doorstep and sending me messages of love and...well, I felt OK. Not on top of the world, of course: a little tired and fuzzy headed, with constantly watering eyes and nose and a tickly cough, and becoming ever more impatient with food tasting like bicarbonate of soda diluted with muddy water – but other than that, I could function pretty well.

That was Epirubicin.

The following three sessions of Taxotere took me by surprise. Suddenly the tickly cough had developed into a keep-everyone-not-to-mention-yourself-awake hacking cough, AKA *chemo cough*. It remained in place for the next nine weeks of treatment and mercifully finally drifted away two weeks after my final chemo session. Then there was the onset of *restless legs syndrome*, the condition which sounds little worse than a severe case of busyness but which is in fact quite debilitating and certainly all-consuming. The legs become overcome with a sort of tingly, twitchy, insect-crawling sensation from which the only relief is to shake or thump the leg, or jump or hop on the spot, much to the amusement of your family. Not so amusing in the middle of the night, however, when you'd rather not jump out of your warm bed to perform a dance routine – a soundless dance routine – for fear of waking your partner from his few moments of sleep gained in the rare break from your chemo cough.

And oh, how my bones and muscles ached, like they'd been put inside a vice and the torturer just wouldn't stop squeezing.

So I wasn't sleeping.

And when I was awake, I couldn't eat because everything still tasted of the delightful mud and bicarbonate of soda recipe. It's amazing how much taste is linked to appetite and how much appetite is linked to your ability to eat. It sounds obvious doesn't it? But wouldn't you think that if you knew you had to eat, if you were hungry, if you normally liked your food and some kind person had placed a piece of warm toast in front of you, that you would be able to eat it? Often I would manage a slice, but only after ten minutes of chewing the MDF, chipboard mix. Something happens to your salivary glands as well I'm afraid, making food seem very dry and thus difficult to chew. And I had a mouthful, truly a mouthful, of ulcers and bleeding gums. At first I could pass the food between the ulcers but after a while, all routes became barred.

But keep reading because help is available.

When I filled out my questionnaire about the three weeks which had followed my first dose of Taxotere, I was in trouble with the nurses. Why had I suffered without calling them? I shouldn't have let things get so bad. But I couldn't think what they could have done, it just had to be 'got through,' didn't it? No!

For my aching bones I was prescribed a lower dose of the injections to boost the bone marrow's creation of white blood cells which are depleted by chemo, and that made an enormous difference. The achiness is part caused by the chemo, but also your over-worked bone marrow complaining about its increased workload. For the other aggravations I came away with a carrier bag full of medications including anaesthetic for my mouth, Laxido for my poor turgid bowels, eye drops for the gritty sensation in my eyes and an average year's dose of painkillers. Although I can't pretend my magic carrier bag took away all of the side-effects, I never had another night crying on the bathroom floor in the early hours, wishing I could just be taken to hospital, sedated and woken a few weeks later when the chemo had stopped and the side-effects had disappeared.

My Mum was a nurse and I was brought up being told that the first course of action for any illness was to have a drink. It was tea, generally, back in the 80s. Unfortunately my badly-done-by new millennium children only get offered water in this type of situation. Sleep was next, and only when the potential for both those remedies had been exhausted could we possibly consider the medical route. Before I had cancer I'd continued much the same. A box of paracetamol would be out of date before I'd used them all. Ibuprofen? Best to keep them in reserve in case one day I'd need them to ease an unexpected amputation. I've since learnt that there are no medals for suffering in silence and I'd advise taking any assistance offered to you. Ask the ward staff, your Key Worker or Breast Cancer Nurse, your oncologist or your GP what can be done.

Don't forget to look at holistic symptom relief, too. I used to suffer with water retention in my stomach and ankles when I was being treated with chemo and Herceptin which, physically and mentally, made me feel very sluggish. Reflexology eased the problem. My six free sessions were provided by the Sir Robert Ogden Macmillan Centre at Harrogate Hospital. I was also about to start a course in ear acupuncture to combat the hot sweats which come with chemo and Tamoxifen, but by then my flushes had already calmed down enormously.

Mindfulness, an ancient Buddhist practice which can work wonders in calming a frantic mind in today's busy world, can help with anything from needle anxiety to coping with The Fear which overwhelms us all sometimes. Your General Practice or hospital may run mindfulness sessions and courses are widely available both through cancer charities and private organisations.

Remember that chemo doesn't last forever and it's unusual for the side-effects to be unbearable for the entire three weeks between treatments. In my experience the effect was cumulative, however, and the weeks coping with previous chemo sessions took their toll on my energy levels and resistance. So be kind to yourself. Just because you feel much better on day fourteen after your first chemo, doesn't mean you have to jump up and clean the windows with a toothbrush, or chair a board meeting of demanding senior executives. Unless you want to of course, in which case you should pounce on the opportunity just as soon as you're ready to be up and at 'em.

Chemo brain

If you've ever had, or been around anyone who's had, a touch of the Pregnancy Brain or its natural rite of passage, New Baby Mush, then you are on the way to understanding the effects of Chemo Brain. Just magnify the lack of cognitive skills, difficulty in concentrating beyond the fourth word in any sentence, and lack of recall for anything which happened approximately ten seconds ago, and you start to get the picture.

I'm not your archetypal control freak. I yearn for those moments where I can grab a back seat because somebody else has taken the reins. But I do like a certain control in my personal and working life because the moment it gets a little messy my to-do list ramps up the stress levels. Chemo Brain certainly added a layer of stress to my life and I think that if you asked my children what the worst aspect of my treatment was, they'd say it was having a Mum who was away with the fairies. I couldn't retain even the most simple of information – from whether I'd brought in the milk to where my children were. Lists, always a big feature of my life, helped me muddle through.

Coping with chemo

Lots of people will give you advice on how to cope with cancer treatment but I would simply suggest that you allow yourself to deal with it in the way which suits you best, wherever possible. Most of the time I still ran around like a centipede on heat, but that's because it worked for me. People kindly gave and loaned me magazines and DVDs and although I had every intention of indulging my sedentary side (in fact, I'd secretly looked forward to it), I quickly worked out that sitting still didn't make me happy. Some people enjoy a steady stream of guests but I learnt that I didn't. I preferred to be alone when the side-effects were at their worst and then emerge from the comfort of my home when I was feeling better again. There's no joy for me in being with people when I can't contribute to conversations or laugh with them. And I feel guilty when busy people spend their time looking after me. It took me two treatment cycles to realise that being totally anti-social was acceptable to other people; they just wanted me to do what I needed to do. Maybe this is a time in your life when you can be a little selfish? Decide what works for you and endeavour to make that happen.

During my three treatment cycle of Taxotere there were days when I had to admit defeat. My ever-slowing editing finally ground to a halt. I stopped trying to write emails when I couldn't remember to whom I needed to respond or about what I was replying.

I read more novels. I even watched some of Wimbledon – live, not the half-hour of highlights when I'd already heard the results four times over, or the Radio Five commentary while I cooked tea, sorted out the washing and waited on hold for telephone banking simultaneously. The last time I'd watched a match in its entirety was about 30 years before.

Be kind to yourself. When you're having chemo, you're allowed to be kind to yourself. This is one of the reasons why having chemo is not all bad.

Once you start to feel better, you tend to improve very quickly and it would be unusual to regress before the next cycle, unless of course, you have an infection and then you must contact the hospital immediately. So don't be afraid to start making arrangements to leave the four walls of your home just as soon as you feel able. I used to clear my diary from day three after my dose of chemo until day ten, and make sure I'd organised some treats to look forward to during the final week before my next chemo when I knew I'd feel at my best.

Fighting Cancer, Living Life

This might have been little more than a cappuccino – or two – with friends, but when you've lost your appetite and energy to chemo and they return for a three-day-teaser, that coffee and a giggle can be magical.

I don't know if this is usual but in the week running up to chemo, I felt a pressing urge to sort out the disorderly disarray which had descended upon my house. I felt fit again. My taste buds would be almost working normally and the sore mouth not so sore, certainly well enough to sip a cup of tea (and thus all was right with the world). The renewed energy inclined me to jump up and sing, but also to clean my cupboards, organise my email stream, sort the finances and clear out the washing basket. I would thus venture into my next chemo with a vague sense of order and somehow that made the few days of total ineffectiveness which would inevitably follow much easier to bear.

I wouldn't have chosen to have chemo, obviously, but the process itself was far from awful. Each treatment was another step further on towards recovery and I ticked them off like this:

Number one: first one done.

Two down: we're a third of the way through.

Three already: we're half way there.

Chemo four: I've done more sessions than I've got left to do.

Chemo five: the next one will be my last.

Six: well, in three weeks' time I won't have to come back to hospital for chemo. In fact, God and powers-that-be willing, I may never have to have chemo again.

Your Personality in Your Hands

The road through Cancerville was a little rocky last week. However sure I was that I didn't want to use the much documented Cold Cap, and however prepared I felt for my hair falling out, the speed with which it all disappeared was shocking. In three days it was pretty much gone. What feels like chunks of your personality falling out in handfuls can only be described as very distressing. The seventy year old man I glimpsed whenever I had the misfortune to catch myself in the mirror, or reflection in a window, was not a sight which gladdened my heart.

But, like those before me and those who will unfortunately follow, I have come through the other side and am starting to embrace life with a bald head; a very cold bald head.

Now I feel able to say to anyone going through this, or holding the hand of someone who is, don't feel you have to pretend that losing your hair is OK, because it isn't. You don't have to tell yourself you look better bald, unless you do. But do remember that hair loss due to chemo is only temporary. For some little understood reason, hair often starts to grow back in cycle four of chemo, not weeks after the end of the final cycle as I'd imagined. And that means that in six small weeks, we could be seeing some tufts of new growth and wondering what colour the baby hair will be (anything but Silver Fox for me, please). Will it be curly or straight? If I get a dose of chemo curl to add to my natural curl, I'll have an 'afro', something which would gain me great kudos with my teenage children. If I go straight, finally I'll have the sophisticated 'together' look us curly-haired mops can never quite pull off. Alas, I fear suave sophistication doesn't come as a package but a first impression of decorum wouldn't go amiss.

When I went out for the first time with my wig on, it felt like I was wearing a sandwich board broadcasting the artificial nature of my head covering to all and sundry. But it doesn't anymore. Wearing a Buff (a sporty headscarf) to the gym felt like I was screaming, 'Caution! Poorly person on treadmill!' Albeit in reality, some people smiled, others gave me a hug and most people didn't notice.

The pain of last week's hair loss feels a lot further away.

Losing your hair

When I originally wrote about chemo and its effect on hair, I only concerned myself with its falling out. After six months of living with baldness and another six of growing my hair back, I now have so much more to say.

With my shorter cut, my wig ready to go and the continual voice in my head telling me that my hair style was stuck in a time-warp anyway, I thought I'd prepared well for my hair's evacuation. Alas, I now realise that you can't fully prepare yourself for losing your hair in these circumstances. The speed with which my hair departed was shocking and for the first time since the very early days of diagnosis, I cried as I held clumps of my hair in my hands. As much as anything, it was a physical representation of the reality of Cancerville, but like everything involved in this process, time helped me to come to terms with it.

How fast did it happen? I noticed clumps of hair in my hands as I washed it on a Monday, the 17th March to be precise, but there was no more after I'd finished washing my hair. I laughed to myself. I'd imagined it! The next day, exactly two weeks after my first dose of chemo, which is pretty standard, the hair filled the basin of the shower and there was no denying it any more. On Wednesday I had my new bob cut to a 'boy's style'. I can't pretend I liked it but I told myself it would make it easier to kiss it goodbye. By Thursday you could see my scalp, Friday I was wearing a wig and by Saturday it had all gone – which was pretty damn quick. Some people keep some hair through their second and even third or fourth treatments. I guess I might have clung on to a few sprouts of frazzled hair but actually, the sight of Saturday's bald head with its few tufts was not one to behold and my husband duly did the honours of shaving off the last strands. There, he said, a perfect head.

People always tell you that you have a perfect head. I think they'd have told me that if I'd had a bald-scape of craters and rock pools, but nonetheless, it was somewhat of a comfort to know that no horrors had been lurking underneath my thirty plus years of dense, curly frizziness. I say only 30 years because my hair first went curly when I was 14. I had wondered if the process might be reversed this time round.

It's staggering how much hair we have on our heads. I had eight inches cut off mine in preparation for chemo, leaving behind a chin length bob. On the first real day of loss, when I could have filled a small carrier bag with the stuff, I went to a parents' evening, feeling incredibly self-conscious, only to find that nobody appeared to be able to tell. Or were they just being polite? I asked one of my closest friends who said that she had just been thinking what great condition my hair was in.

I'm delighted to say that my concerns for mounds of hair on my pillow and all over my clothes went unfounded and I may have had a hand in that. I learnt that when hair is going to fall out it will fall out. You can try hair-saving measures such as not washing it, going easy on the products and certainly not using any heat to dry or straighten it. But it's like trying to repair a hole in the roof with a piece of Sellotape; it's only ever going to be a temporary measure.

I was surprised to see that where some areas of hair had come loose, others were still stuck firm. Indeed, I found that a good few handfuls of hair would fall out and then the process would stop for a few hours; even if I tugged at the hair (not recommended), it didn't come away. Thus, I got into the ritual of leaning over the toilet (my apologies for the image but there's nothing glamorous about your hair falling out) and gently massaging my scalp. The emphasis is on 'gently'. I massaged every loose strand into the pan, and no doubt clogged up the pipes. I should probably recommend you lean over a waste paper basket.

Massaging to release the loosened wisps meant that once accomplished, I could leave the house knowing that any remaining locks would be in place for the next few hours. Repeat the process before bedtime and I could wake up in the morning looking almost the same as the night before, and crucially having avoided the 'hairy pillow' I so feared. It's funny the ridiculous things we worry about when we have cancer but my disdain for the hairy pillow and hairy clothing was a big deal to me. I wonder if it's because the world of Cancerville into which we've been plunged is one without control and with little sense of order, so snatches of normality can take on huge importance.

Something else I found through first-hand experience was how sore the scalp can be when you're losing your hair in this perverse, time-lapse film kind of way. So the massage technique was a very pleasant experience, providing great relief to the soreness which I can only describe as being like sunburn to the scalp. Those of you who have ever been bald on a surprisingly hot summer's day, will know the feeling I'm describing.

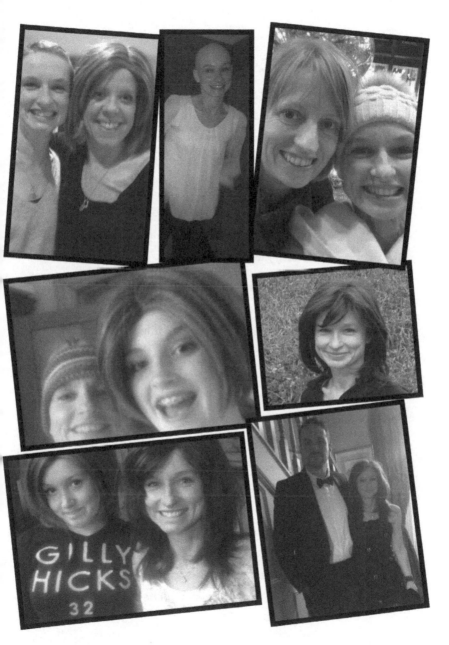

Fighting Cancer, Living Life

The wig phase

Wearing a wig was quite good fun, perhaps because I had three. I had one for 'day wear', one for 'going out' and one for 'a change'. Being various lengths and versions of sleek and straight, all my wigs were entirely different to the hair I'd left behind, and I enjoyed looking a little different for the first time in my adult life.

By the way, prepare to 'lose' your wig to your friends and family constantly. There is something infectious about wearing a wig. Everybody wants to try it on.

There's a huge range of wigs and a big difference in price. Top of the range are ones made from real hair which have the tremendous advantage of being 'stylable'. They can be washed, dried, curled, straightened, or anything that you can do with normal hair, in fact. Go for synthetic and there's none of that and in addition, you have to watch sudden propulsions of heat such as opening the oven door, or standing too close to a boiling kettle. The ends can quickly singe leaving your proud new locks looking like those of a neglected Barbie doll. I'd also say that synthetic wigs have a fairly short shelf life. By the end of its stint, the ends of my 'everyday' wig were looking rather split and like I was a few months overdue a cut. That said it pretty much lasted as long as I needed it to last. It feels discourteous and incredibly ungrateful to say this, as very kind souls donate several inches of their hair to help make up real-hair wigs. But in the interests of decision making, I will say that I personally struggled a little with the concept of wearing someone else's hair on my head. I also had to keep asking which of the wigs I was trying were real hair and which were synthetic. Artificial wigs can be amazingly life-like and are not to be confused with the fancy dress versions. If I couldn't tell the difference between real and fake, I figured even those in close proximity would also struggle. It meant I had carte blanche to choose the type I was most comfortable with – cost notwithstanding. I chose a mid-range, synthetic wig, which became my go-to wig, the one I'd wear most of the time. With that came a fairly advanced mesh base which cunningly looked like my scalp peeking through if anyone got too close. You see, there are all these things we don't think about until forced, who'd have thought that the colour of our scalp affected the appearance of our hair? Too pale and your head looks like it's been painted with undercoat, too dark and it looks like you're wearing a wig over sunburn.

One more tip. There is something about a synthetic wig in flash photography which doesn't work. Somehow it picks up the light differently and fills its wearer with abject panic, thinking that all the time they'd been told that nobody would ever know they had artificial locks, it was a lie of Emperor's new Clothes proportions. It isn't. The camera is lying in this instance. And if you're wondering how I can be so sure that my friends' reassurances were built on truth rather than kindness, one of my best friends was diagnosed with breast cancer four months after me (I know) and let's just say that her wig looked totally authentic in real life...

I bought my main wig with my NHS grant for which I had to pay a set fee. It's currently £65 but obviously that figure might change. Grants for wigs are also available through the Macmillan cancer charity, **Macmillan.org.uk**. Since my wig wearing days I've heard of a wonderful charity called Wigbank (**www.wigbank.com**) which takes second hand wigs of all varieties and prices and, after a thorough cleaning, sells them for a fraction of their original cost.

One kind soul donated me her wig from when she'd had breast cancer five years previously and the third I bought in a wig sale. Yep, suddenly I was trawling the internet for bargain wigs and discovering a range of companies I'd never have known existed. **https://www.naturalimagewigs.co.uk/** and **http://www.hothair.co.uk** are where I spent most time.

Something to consider when buying a wig is that it will need washing with a special wig shampoo every few wears, and it takes a good 12 to 24 hours for it to dry. Some people interchange their wig wearing with scarves, and others only wear their wigs on certain occasions, but if you think you may be someone who'll wear a wig every day, a second one would be very useful.

Wigs and sport don't go together so you might need to consider an alternative if you're the energetic type. I used to run in a bandana and this brand is both UV- protected and breathable so is particularly comfortable: **www.buffwear.co.uk.**

Everybody asks you if you're worried the wig will blow off unexpectedly. But no, mine never did, and even walking along blustery coastlines I never felt that it would. I declined a rollercoaster ride on an exceedingly blustery day once, and stayed below deck on a particularly windy ferry journey, as I thought these extreme scenarios might have seen me pushing my luck, but otherwise, wigs tend to sit firm. You wear an attractive little piece of hosiery underneath – pretty similar to what you'd wear if you were going to rob a bank – which acts like a sort of scalp superglue.

The wig stayed put even when I was being spun around by a friend at a ball who was performing some impressively energetic jive routines. This was much to the distress of his wife who was convinced he'd forgotten I was wearing a wig and was dreading the moment when it would fly across the room, perch itself atop the baldest of male guests, and be forever enshrined as a YouTube moment worthy of a few million clicks. In fact, my major concern that evening was the heat. I was so hot with the high impact aerobics style dancing and synthetic covered scalp, that I could have happily pulled off my wig and flung it across the room myself.

Happily, I didn't. We can perhaps thank my lack of inebriation for that.

To wig or not to wig

On reflection I would say that our hair is so closely linked to our identity that it isn't surprising that these steps on the way to losing and regaining hair take on such significance. My advice would simply be to go at your own pace and do whatever you need to do with your head to make you most comfortable.

I know people who have never worn a wig, who've embraced the smooth and perfect scalp look and pulled it off brilliantly. But that wasn't for me. Others would wear wigs in public but greeted the postman bald and proud; it was their home after all. That wasn't for me either. But I did have a great selection of hats I could slip on if the doorbell went as they were quicker to don than a wig, so I was never caught out.

I know others who chose scarves instead of wigs but I couldn't find a scarf I liked. They made me feel old and as though I was making more of a statement about having cancer than I wanted to make. I've always been more than happy to talk about my plight but I liked to feel in control of who knew. I didn't want a stranger in a queue to give me an inquisitive stare or even one of sympathy, or a small child to ask their parent in a room-silencing voice why I had no hair.

But that's me. And that isn't to say that scarves don't suit other people. They are cooler, more versatile and certainly cheaper – you could have a drawer full for the price of one wig. Your local hospital or cancer centre will undoubtedly hold a free session where you can try on an array of different styles. Wig shops also stock a range of scarves and hair pieces, too.

These companies also seem to have a good reputation and range: **http://www.suburbanturban.co.uk/women-hair-loss/winter-hats/womens-hair-loss-chemo-winter-hat-esther/** and **http://www.annabandana.co.uk/**

It's not just your head

Where the wig covered bald head wasn't as bad as I thought it might be, other hair loss was more difficult. Literature focuses on losing the hair on our head but trust me, it goes a lot lower than that.

And then there are the eyebrows and eyelashes. Not everybody loses them, apparently, but I have yet to meet anyone being treated with chemo for breast cancer who didn't lose at least some of their lashes and brows. I lost all my eye lashes and only clung on to a couple of clumps of eyebrow hair which were neither use nor ornament.

I found this hard. Being bald doesn't actually make you look poorly, or even older, in my experience, but having lash-less eyes, particularly when they're constantly streaming with the very common, watery-eyed, side-effect of chemo and Herceptin, does. And I hadn't appreciated quite how much we need our eyebrows to frame our face. Simply put, with my bald head I looked like Jackie without hair. With my bald face, I didn't look like me, I looked like somebody else who could do with a good month or so of sleep, not to mention a few dozen portions of fruit and veg and a long holiday in the sun.

But please don't despair. All this hair grows back eventually. Even the hair on your legs, which is a bit of a shame as mine had never been so smooth. My eyelashes and eyebrows started to return around three months after the end of chemo and putting my first mascara on a couple of months later made me whoop with delight.

A warning, though: patience is required. The growing back takes a while and can have a slightly haphazard approach. I had to stick my new eyebrow hairs down with eyebrow 'glue', insistent as they were in growing at right angles to my face. My eyebrows are still very patchy and my eyelashes are short but it's progress and there are lots of little tricks and tools to help smooth the way, not least a bulging make-up bag, most of which I got for free from the Look Good, Feel Good session at my local hospital (see **http://www.lookgoodfeelbetter.co.uk**). **Macmillan.org.uk** runs similar events in conjunction with Boots advisors, and I've also managed to snag a place at a No.7 make-up demonstration, complete with goody bag, at my local Haven in Leeds.

For a more lasting solution, there are 'semi-permanent make-up' options such as an eyebrow tattoo service which is often heavily subsidised, or even free, to people who've gone through cancer treatment. I had discounted eyelash extensions, and although I couldn't afford to have them done at full price, they did make me feel a little more human at a time when it was proving challenging to coat mascara on my five single lashes. There are many different places offering the service and there's lots of information online. This blog taught me a lot: **http://www.beautydespitecancer.co.uk/beauty/all-about-brows**

Hair and parabens

After my first 'new growth hair wash' with baby shampoo –
keep reading – desperate for my hair to grow several inches
overnight, every night, I sought advice. I booked myself into
the hospital's 'hair clinic', a voluntary run session specifically
for people who've lost their hair to chemo. Most hospitals
and many charities such as The Haven run similar sessions.
My visit was in early September, around the time I posted on
Facebook that I'd measured 4mm of hair on my head. I still
had my hair covered by my wig at that stage, but nonetheless,
considered it to be oh so long.

To be honest, I didn't really think the hairdresser would be able
to tell me much. It wasn't as if having hair was new to me,
right? Wrong! Maureen's opening gambit was to suggest that
I'd used baby shampoo.

Correct.

Bad idea, she said.

Maureen explained that baby shampoo was actually not kind
to hair at all. Its primary objective was not to sting babies'
eyes. It achieved that brilliantly but at a chemical price.
Chemicals which took away the sting also stripped the hair of
its health.

I was interested in this. I'd decided that as I'd been forced to
lose my trademark bird's nest, cultivated over many years of

neglect in the form of cheap products and an over-indulgence in gooey serums to tame the Michael Jackson look, I would use this as an opportunity to grow a healthier mane second time around. And fast, please. Decision one: no more baby shampoo for me.

Are you washing your hair every day? Maureen asked. I knew the answer to this one. Gosh no! I didn't want to strip it of its lovely baby-ness. Wrong again! Maureen said that shampoo only stripped the hair of its goodness if you used cheap products. Daily washing kept the scalp clean and promoted a healthy environment for the hair to grow. It was a bit like soil. Healthy plants needed healthy roots which needed healthy soil. Moreover, if I really wanted to look after my hair, and health, I should consider paraben-free products. It made sense but I was still a little sceptical. Hair grows as hair grows, surely? A little quicker for some and slower for others, but generally at a rate of a quarter of an inch per month, as Mr Google suggested.

Still, I gratefully accepted the handful of additive-free samples and agreed to try Maureen's system. I was to wash and condition my hair every day with the tiniest dollop of this shampoo and conditioner. The shampoo would clean my scalp as well as the hair follicles, encouraging quicker hair growth.

I can only say that my hair absolutely flourished. People I saw on a weekly basis laughed when they saw me, my hair was growing at such an astonishing rate. What's more, my single samples of paraben-free shampoo and conditioner both lasted the whole week of daily washing.

Even as the wife of a man who doesn't wash his hair (which isn't half as bad as it sounds) and who has plentiful, well-conditioned locks, I was starting to think that there might be some science behind the rapid growth formula, even if the logical part of my brain was struggling with the concept. Lush tresses might be attainable, it seemed, but at a significantly higher price than my frizzy mane had cost. Did the lovely Maureen have a stake in hair products costing well over double figures? And what was a paraben anyway, had somebody decided they could play a role in cancer?

Parabens are preservatives used in cosmetic products. They slow the growth of fungus and bacteria and thus prolong the products' life. Maureen had originally bought into the idea of paraben-free hair products when she first owned a salon with her husband in the Eighties. He was suffering allergic reactions and having breathing issues as he worked and she decided to look into the products they were using. Convinced his work environment was the cause, she switched the salon to paraben-free products and his ailments disappeared almost instantly. I'm not usually one for fads and scares but the link Maureen had discovered sounded very plausible to me. Maureen's salon has been paraben-free ever since. She continued to follow the research into parabens and later stumbled across reports of their potential link with cancer.

Really? My oncologist hadn't heard of it. I decided to do my own research. The NHS website **http://www.nhs.uk/news/2012/01January/Pages/parabens-in-breast-cancer-tissue-studied.aspx** explained that a very small study of the breasts of 40 women with cancer following mastectomy, but before they'd been treated with chemo or radiotherapy, showed parabens to be present in the breast tissue. However, the study didn't test the tissue of a healthy breast which may also have shown traces of parabens. The research therefore couldn't state that parabens cause breast cancer, simply that parabens were present in the tissue tested. The most that has been concluded from the study is that parabens can enter the blood stream. The suggestion is that they may enter via our scalp when using hair products or into the breast tissue via the armpit when using deodorants containing parabens. Cancer Research UK, my go-to place for sense-checking scares, states that there is, 'no good scientific evidence' to show that, 'chemicals in common products such as cosmetics or toiletries could raise the risk of cancer.'

I wasn't surprised to read this. There never will be a single product or way of living which we can hold directly responsible for cancer, alas. Otherwise we could all stop doing it, eating it or using it and cancer would be packed off right where it deserves to be, somewhere between hell and a worse place, rubbing shoulders with The Plague and Small Pox.

But something about chemicals getting into my blood via my head didn't sit easily with me either. I'm all for eliminating aspects of my life which *may* play a role in the formation of cancer, particularly if their elimination would have no or little detrimental effect on my lifestyle. These are the best remedies; the easy ones. The more changes I can make in my post-cancer life, the more it helps my confidence that I might inadvertently get it right so that cancer hasn't got a chance should it dare to come calling again.

However, I don't have a bottomless purse so I asked Maureen how much extra she was forced to charge her customers after the switch to paraben-free products. Nothing, she said. She didn't put up her prices at all. She realised that the extra cost was off-set by the dosage: products which weren't pumped with water did the job with a fraction of the amount. The net cost was the same. This is certainly true. Even though my hair is nowhere near the dizzy lengths of yesteryear, I am nonetheless using a pea size amount of product as opposed to the two handfuls I was using of my 3 for 2 off the shelf products from leading supermarkets in the past.

There are various paraben-free brands on offer. The one I stuck with is cheaper than most and if sourced on the internet, compares well with the price of supermarket products. I bought one litre bottles of shampoo and conditioner nine months ago and still have some left.

My hair will never be super glossy and luscious. It's too thick and curly for that. But it is so much softer than it ever used to be and although I am impatient to rid myself of the short crop, I do like the fact that it looks healthier. I think it's safe to say that I am a convert. And my piggy bank is no poorer for it.

Heightened Sensitivity

The trouble with cancer is it's always there; scratching away, nails on the blackboard, a dog barking in the middle of the night or the wind rattling the windows when you've just watched a horror film. It's just *there* – first thing in the morning, last thing at night, meddling, fidgeting in your brain. Will there be more cancer? It asks. Hopefully not. They got rid of the original little pest and the chemo, radiotherapy, Herceptin and Tamoxifen – the wonderful medical people are throwing everything they've got at it – is the belt and braces to keep the little blighter away for good, I tell myself. Excellent, my grey matter responds. But then my irrational self rears its ugly little head and off we go again, Will there be more cancers...? You get the drift.

However, there is a flip side to 'cancer noise' and I can only call it a heightened sensitivity.

The first weekend after results day, my oh–so-supportive hubbie and I went for a walk. We've done this walk several times. Local people will know it as the Fewston and Swinsty reservoirs walk. We first did it with babes in slings, then rucksacks, then prams (I use the plural as I had to return one which fell apart in just a year, only to be told that prams weren't really meant for walking with children but for loading into cars. But that's another story). We did it again with their little legs skipping behind, for a short while with their long legs skipping in front, and now...well they tend to have better things to do.

So, it was just me and him walking a walk we'd walked several times before. Funny, I thought. I've never noticed the smell of the peaty path quite so keenly before. Forgive the cliché but there was a glint of sun over the ripples on the lake and I thought it was mesmerising. Children laughing always makes me smile – isn't that just the nicest of sounds? – but that day it made me beam. And then we went for a cup of tea. It was just a cup of tea in a refurbished pub on a cold day with a loud, crackling fire and candles oozing lavender and jasmine flickering atmospherically. That cup of tea was the most wonderful cup of tea I'd ever drunk. And I drink a lot so that's a pretty bold statement. And so it goes on. I can't really explain it. It's just that when people say nice things to me or others, I really, really notice. When people crack a joke, it's very, very funny. When a song comes on the radio which I love it makes me cry. But it's ok, it's just 'happy to be alive' tears.

And all those moments, which happen several times a day, well, they blot out the cancer noise too.

I hope I appreciated these things before.

Put on the Spot

On an unnaturally hot, Wimbledon Finals Day last June, hubbie and I popped out on a bike ride. We noticed that there was an unfeasibly large amount of cyclists on the road with us and very little traffic. It was only when we spotted that all the other cyclists were wearing event numbers, that we realised we'd become caught up in the annual White Rose Classic cycle event in Yorkshire.

This has happened to us once before. We'd snuck off for a birthday weekend in The Lakes for some champagne and cycling. On a bitterly cold Sunday morning, we clicked into our pedals and marvelled at how many other people had also decided that this rain spattered day was a good opportunity for a bike ride.

I was slightly surprised to be passing quite a few of the other cyclists. I wouldn't bet on me to pass people uphill. As I was overtaking someone, we got chatting about how wonderful it was that so many people were out on their bikes whatever the weather and that this was indeed a bit of a hill, before I was forced to bid my farewell explaining that I needed to catch up with my husband. You go! he said, You're doing so well!

I thought that was very kind of him; I'd only left the B&B thirty minutes previously. It was only when I rounded a corner at the top of the hill to a groundswell of animated cheering and, Go girl! that I clocked all the other cyclists' numbers and realised that we'd inadvertently joined the infamous Fred Whitton Challenge. With its 110 miles over hill and pass, it's generally considered the toughest bike ride in Britain. Everybody else had already done approximately 60 miles of hills and all but the most elite of bikers, were starting to feel it a little. I, however, after my big breakfast and a short warm up, was flying. Indeed, I was first woman past that point, according to the cheering crowd.

However, after laughing so much about my moment of glory, we realised that we were cycling in the wrong direction and the only option was to turn around and cycle back past the bemused crowed. I kept my head down.

Back to the White Rose Classic and a decision to do the race properly on 29th June 2014. Then I got cancer. Chemo has chopped me off at the knee caps a few times but not too often. The rest of the time I've been trip-trapping along in trainers or on pedals, enjoying the wind or sun on my face, plotting challenges. I decided I was still going to give the White Rose a shot – a very slow, last one over the line kind of shot – but I kept it secret in case I was forced to pull out. I really didn't want to let anyone down.

Race day was approaching when a sympathetic nurse told me that my white cell count was low and I'd have to have a

Fighting Cancer, Living Life

re-test before deciding if chemo would go ahead a few days later. I supposed that meant that I shouldn't go for a fifty mile training bike ride that weekend. It surprised me to learn that there's very little you can do to increase, or even decrease, your white cell count. It's just down to how quickly your body manufactures the replacement cells for those lost to the cancer treatment. So, the only problem mixing cycling and chemo was if you had an accident. I could end up in hospital with my body struggling to fight the infection. I didn't like the sound of an infection. I know about efforts to unnaturally encourage my bone marrow to make extra white cells to deal with infection, and the process hurt every bone in my body, even my jaw. I also didn't like the idea that chemo would be halted while the clever people at the hospital patched me back together again.

But the sun was shining and my bike was looking at me like a dog when you've mentioned a walk. Should I categorically not cycle? I asked, one final time. Not necessarily, was the surprising response, but I should consider how likely it was that I'd fall off.

I thought of putting my arm in the spin drier and smashing it into too many pieces to count. I remembered my sky dive over a plant pot which resulted in a broken knee, and I winced at the memory of the pain I felt when I broke my foot twisting it on an embedded tree root whilst running.

Pretty likely to fall off, I thought.

Now, I know cycling isn't for everyone but me? I was disappointed. Gutted. My secret White Rose Challenge was off. Scheduled for twelve days after my penultimate chemo, my white blood cells would be at their lowest. It just wasn't worth it, everyone said.

And then I saw it. I clocked the poster at the local sports centre: Four Hour Spinathon for Marie Curie Cancer Care. A cycling event to raise money for a cancer charity? It had my name written all over it. Yes, me being me, there was still every chance I could fall off my bike during the four class challenge, an exhaustion induced, away-with-the-fairies type of incident, but it would be onto a clean-ish gym floor and with twelve other participants and an instructor on hand to pick me up.

No matter that I haven't actually done any spinning for about six months.

Brilliant, my friend said, I'll do it, too. Well, actually, after she'd had a couple of glasses of wine I told her she'd love it, glossing quickly over the fact that you could choose how many of the four classes you'd like to attempt. Hey! The bigger the challenge, the larger the euphoria at the end!

My other friend I snagged when she was hosting twelve people for an evening of tapas.

So, we've signed up. Those who know me well will understand that arriving on time for the start of a spin class would be an achievement in itself.

Tutu's ready? And we're off!

After 240 minutes on a bike (zero miles travelled) and with four bottles of energy drink, four litres of water, two jelly babies, five Nutella sandwiches and a handful of cashew nuts behind me, I'd completed the four hour Spinathon in aid of Marie Curie Cancer Care **http://www.mariecurie.org.uk/**

It was a great way to spend a morning, even if I did scowl a little at seeing 6am on a Saturday. Wonderful pedalling camaraderie and mad teachers made it fantastic fun and the promised chocolate cake and bucks fizz at the end gave us truly professional athletes that final kick of motivation to keep us going.

The organisers had hoped that the 20 of us who took part in Saturday's Spinathon might raise a good £500. The latest total is in excess of £2,700. We were all overwhelmed and so touched by the support.

Race for Life

I have run the Race for Life several times. I even admit to once coming second, although the girl ahead of me beat me by a whopping three minutes so please don't be too impressed. When I'd run it too many times to ask for sponsorship again, I decided to marshal the run and then I spent the next few years running it with my children, painfully dragging my youngest round when she was tiny.

It only seemed appropriate that in June 2014, I should run the race again with my girls. But I was struggling before I'd even put on my kit. I'd just had my final dose of Taxotere, the chemo renowned for achy bones and tired muscle syndrome. It was an effort even to lift up my feet. I finished the run crying, granted because my eyes were constantly streaming on chemo, but also because the achievement felt as great as running a marathon. I crossed the line with my bandana covering my bald head and a note on my back saying that I was running in sadness for my friends who have been taken too soon by cancer (pancreatic, stomach cancer and brain tumour) and in gratitude for my mother-in-law (lymphoma and breast cancer twice), my brother-in-law and dear friend (both testicular cancer) and one of my very best friends who was diagnosed with breast cancer four months after I was (you couldn't make it up).

And I was running – well, shuffling – for me, for all of us lucky ones. I was pushed over the line by the cheers of the generous crowd and with the amusement of my teenage daughters who have known me finish races late because I've got lost, but not because my legs wouldn't budge. I felt such an enormous sense of achievement. I'd recommend it to anyone. Doing something for charity and being active do make you feel better. It's as simple as that. It really doesn't matter what speed you run. Remember to ask for sponsorship, though. The organisers, the wonderful Cancer Research UK, are totally reliant on fundraising as they receive no government funding for their work.

For all those whose sporting life has taken a bashing from cancer treatment, hang on in there. A year later, I ran the Race for Life with my children again. I didn't shuffle the 5k but ran the 10k. It was good to be back and another reminder that treatment doesn't go on for ever. As soon as it stops, you can get back on with your life.

Sport and exercise

I will never know how I would have felt through chemo and other treatments if I hadn't tried to continue with my usual running and cycling antics, but I can say that I'm glad I tried. I did lose fitness. Where I would usually bound up hill, my legs felt like they were wading through the thickest grass, while sinking into quicksand, and where I would usually cycle twenty miles before even daring to suggest a coffee stop, I was gasping before I'd started the second hill. But having a focus, forcing myself to take in some fresh air, and probably more important than anything, feeling like I hadn't completely lost a sense of self, were godsends to me in the difficult days of treatment. I never went more than a few days without doing any sport, not that you'd know it if you saw me run The Race for Life. Sometimes I'd have to force myself to go and get my trainers, but when I got home after a run or stepped off my bike, I always felt better than before I started. Of course, some days I didn't do anything at all and pottered guilt-free instead around the house. You can justify anything when you're on chemo.

Why Not Me?

I quite expected to get cancer. Even though I prefer my glass most definitely half full, I've always been a, 'Why not me?', rather than a, 'Why me?' kind of girl. I think accepting the unsavoury situations which jump out at us unbidden, is the first step to giving them a great big slap in the chops.

And 1 in 3 people will contract cancer at some point in their life so why wouldn't one of those people be me? I guess I just hoped that I'd be 109 when it knocked and so short on faculties that I wouldn't really notice. But no matter, I'm here, having treatment for cancer and this is how I intend to move forward.

I thank my lucky stars that I developed cancer in 2014 rather than 1974 because the treatment available these days means that chances of survival for most – alas not all – cancers are so much better than when I was growing up, and rising all the time. But treatment is brutal, expensive and not fool-proof and thus prevention would be infinitely preferable.

Whilst the experts know how cancers are formed, they don't always know why one person contracts cancer and another doesn't. Once the well-publicised triggers such as smoking, excessive alcohol, obesity, sun exposure and genetics have been discounted, medicine puts it down to bad luck. In this case we're grateful for the brilliance of modern treatment and hope that we're not unlucky again.

However, this is the one area of science which doesn't work for me. I get twitchy putting my life in the care of luck. The body is clever but cancer cells are evil little blighters. We're back to my, 'Why not me?' scenario. Something about the mix of my body, my diet, my environment, my genetics, even my character meant that I developed cancer. And I cannot see any logic that says that if I change nothing, this won't happen again. I needed an action plan.

But to be able to hatch my plan, I had to understand how cancer was formed.

I shall endeavour to explain it how I understand it, in my — spent longer revising to scrape through (*I reckon it's the easiest science so I'll choose that one*) Biology O-level than all my other subjects put together — kind of way. I apologise in advance to those who know their stamen from their stigma or what the periodic table was actually for.

It's all about cells. I imagine our body like a small town inhabited by cells; a little like an ant colony. There are hospitals equipping white blood cells with the tools to fight infection. There's the train collecting and depositing oxygen around the body so that it functions efficiently and productively. Constant building work is going on to make new bones or repair over-stressed muscles and joints. Then of course there are the big organs made up of lots of cells and commanding great respect. If the body gets over-taxed, the lesser organs are ordered to go into standby to ensure the brain and the heart stay in control and manage the body out of the crisis.

It's a very harmonious town. Yes, things go wrong. The control centre for each cell – its DNA – can become damaged and feed it the wrong instructions so that it becomes a faulty cell and be no use to the body. This happens fairly regularly, it would seem, but these Bad Cells are generally expelled; a very necessary and common process in the body's continual pursuit of good health.

However, the body's defences don't always work as effectively as they should and sometimes a Bad Cell isn't ejected but instead reproduces uncontrollably. Left unchecked (and the body has many checking systems; we are talking a perfect storm here) Bad Cells will eventually grow too powerful for the body's defences. Eventually, our town faces more than a cluster of Bad Cells, instead, it's now a cancerous lump. Now, the most effective tool open to the body is to call in the heavies, the medical profession, who come with a big spade to uproot the lump and cast it from the body forever.

That can be the end of it, but if the cancer has been around for a while or is a particularly fast growing cancer – like mine, many thanks for that, *body* – it might have got cocky and started throwing out baby cancer cells which could be hiding somewhere in the body. Or the lump could have taken root in a very built up, hard to reach area and the spade can't get near it. If there's a chance of this the super powers come in, launching chemo, a bomb which reverberates right around the body. It kills off all fast growing cells such as our hair and disease fighting cells, and within this group of fast growing cells are, you've got it, the fastest growing of them all: cancer cells. See you bad boys! In the super power's army are other fighters such as radiotherapy which attacks locally and the peace keeping forces such as Herceptin and Tamoxifen. These are protein and hormone inhibitors without which some types of breast cancer struggle to divide and conquer, and which hang around long after chemo has done its bit, maintaining the status quo.

So, back to my action plan; what was it that I did to create an environment in which the Bad Cell thrived? Why didn't my defence system work quite as well as it should have done? And the, 'Why not me?' question: why wouldn't this happen again?

I'm quite a healthy soul. I've always loved sport and spend hours every week doing it. Much to the constant consternation of my sisters and friends (I'll whisper it) I don't much care for cake, am happier munching my way through a bowl of salad. So, she says, glossing over the daughter's warm banana cake devoured last night, my diet is naturally fairly healthy. Breast cancer doesn't run in my family. I've never smoked and when it comes to alcohol, I'm generally considered a, 'bit of a lightweight'. But more about that later.

I'm very wary of scare stories and don't tend to trust information unless it's endorsed by recognised cancer charities and bodies. My favourites are Cancer Research UK and Macmillan Cancer Support, not least because I know that stats are 'hidden' on these sites, protecting people like me who don't want to see them. I've read up on diet, environment and the validity and otherwise of well-documented cancer triggers we hear of in the news, and this is what I've come up with. I'm not saying it's a check list of what every person needs to do to prevent cancer or to stop it coming back, nor indeed is it a catch-all list. After all, if it was, I'd be very rich and decorated with various honours, not least the Nobel Prize for Science – and did I mention my lack of aptitude for science? But, in addition to some small diet tweaks, broccoli and walnuts to name but two, here are two changes I've chosen to make based on my own research and lifestyle.

1. **Sleep**

    There has been much in the press about shift workers living less long than day time workers, and there is some evidence that not allowing the body enough time to regenerate can increase the risk of some serious ailments including stroke, obesity, diabetes and, interestingly, the *recurrence* of aggressive breast cancers. This is early research but to see any link at all when I am someone who's rarely slept more than five hours a night since my teens, was enough for me to make a definite change to my sleeping habits. Before midnight is when I now got to bed, seven hours later is when I wake. Much as I lament that with the new regime has come a loss of ten hours of my old writing time every week, I can't write a book from the next life can I?

Well, I don't think I can, anyway.

An unexpected bi-product of this was that after only a few nights of better sleep, people noticed. I recognise that people may have expected me to have grown three noses after my diagnosis but nonetheless, I had many comments on how *well* I looked, including one friend who'd said she'd spotted I'd been looking tired (oh the shame) but she'd put it down to us all getting older. Pah! Forget anti-wrinkle cream, my advice for serious, and not so serious reasons, is that if you're skimping on the zzz, get thee to bed!

2. **Alcohol**

Unfortunately, women drinking any more than 2-3 units of alcohol a day put themselves at a slightly higher risk of developing breast and other cancers. For men the safe limit is 3-4 units. Remember when I said that I was a bit of a lightweight when it came to alcohol? So that was fine, no need to make any changes there. But then I looked into what a unit really is and realised that 2-3 units per day is actually more like **one** standard drink a day. I didn't drink every night of the week pre-cancer, nor did I binge drink before, but I did regularly drink more than one glass of alcohol in one sitting. Now I don't drink more than seven units a week and it's been surprisingly easy to make the shift.

No longer do my husband and I crack open a bottle of wine during the week – it would last us a couple of nights, like I say, we're not talking your classic high risk here – unless we have someone round to supper. If we go out at the weekend, I'll have a glass of wine. It's all I need. I just like that first taste, like the first chocolate: always the best and downhill from there. I like the fact that I can join in a toast for someone's birthday, have a splash of wine in the sun, a glass of red with a Sunday roast, but I also like the fact that I don't wake up next morning with the horrendous sinking feeling that I might have increased my risk of breast cancer.

That said, all the advice I've read and been given in hospital is that these are lifetime choices. Break the rules now and again and the result will not be automatic cancer. Nor will all heavy and even light drinkers get breast cancer. Remember, cancerous cells are the result of a perfect storm, a multitude of ongoing factors, only some of which we can influence.

Please don't have nightmares!

Luck

I don't consider myself unlucky to have got cancer, I call it life. But I do consider it to be very lucky indeed that my Grade 3 primary cancer was caught early, still relatively small but growing fast, and that the goal for the medical profession was cure. It was lucky that the lump was where it was and that it was prominent enough for me to feel it. It's lucky that I live in an age where, thanks to massive funding together with the awe-inspiring cleverness of scientists, breakthroughs in the fight against cancer are happening all the time. I even have hope for my friends with secondaries or grade four breast cancers, supposedly incurable but becoming less incurable all the time.

And I was lucky that a voice in my head told me not to wait a month to see if the lump decreased in size as suggested by my GP. It wasn't her fault. I'd led her down the path of thinking that the lump might have gone down in size during the week of waiting for my appointment. I think I'd just got used to it after the initial knee breaking moment when I'd felt the lump by chance, a few days earlier. That was very lucky indeed.

I am not complacent. And I admit the fear of cancer's return, and that next time I might not be so lucky, does haunt me from time to time.

We are human, we have moments when we look in the mirror and see a bald version of our father, minus the eyebrows, and it all seems just a little bit like hard work. But the rest of the time, we have to rejoice and be grateful. I think it's ungrateful of me to be sad about my lot. My lot was to survive cancer. I am one of the lucky ones and I intend to continue living my life to the full to show my appreciation of that one. Please kick me if I don't.

Control and lifestyle

So, have I kept up my good intentions? You know, I have, largely, yes. The biggest change I needed to make was in my sleep patterns. Given half the chance I would still happily spend my days in a sleepy haze only to wake at 8pm and proceed to stay up all night. Night owl is definitely my natural leaning. I don't do that. I daren't do that. But sometimes the bedtime slips the wrong side of midnight. What I never do now, however, is have two very late nights in a row. I sleep for seven hours most nights of the week, compared to the average of around five hours of sleep a night I'd been managing on since I was a teen.

I've kept to the seven units of alcohol a week maximum I imposed upon myself. My recent discovery of a rosé and sparkling water spritzer has helped. It tastes like weak pink bubbly, is perfect for a sun-soaked summer evening and rolls in at a helpful half the units. Sometimes, not often, I'll push the proverbial boat out and drink four of my allocation of units in one night, but austerity quickly resumes and I abstain the next day and often the next few nights as well. Sometimes I'd like to drink a bit more, or not have to be so conscious of it, but I can't and that's just the way it is. That, I'm afraid, is life.

I'm still eating lots of seeds, walnuts and broccoli. Generally specific diet eliminations and additions (as opposed to eating a healthy, balanced diet) are rejected by the organisations I trust, such as **http://www.cancerresearchuk.org/** and **http:// www.nhs.uk/** , but you know, just in case. And I like them, even broccoli. Because I rarely hear much that's positive about cheap red meat, bacon and other processed meats, I seldom eat them. I'm undecided on the possible link between milk and a hormone receptive breast cancer. One man's disdain for dairy products is another's low calcium levels and potential osteoporosis risk. It's a minefield, isn't it? But as it's clearly not a balanced diet to start the day with a large bowl of cereal and end it the same way, having not found the time to eat seven-a-day-packed-meal I've prepared for the family, I haven't had cereal for dinner since before I found out I had cancer.

Something new

There's another life choice I've considered since my original post which is still a work in progress. But it's an area which I think a lot of us could, and should, consider.

There are some people in life who are totally serene. They move slowly from place to place, talk in a considered manner and have few lines on their forehead. You know the people I mean.

I am not one of them.

But one such lady is the therapist who gave me acupuncture to try to combat the hot flushes that chemo and Tamoxifen kindly deliver.

The therapist and I would chat as the needles went in and once I said how much I loved coming to see her because I got two-for-one: counselling as well as acupuncture. Oh no! she said, you don't need counselling. You know exactly what you need to do, carrying it out is your problem and for that you need life coaching.

The therapist, we'll call her Jane, totally buys into the suggested link between lack of sleep and cancer. Indeed, when we dissected my lifestyle, she considered this to be the biggest factor in my diagnosis. Jane finds me stressful. Even the speed I walk into the room makes her nervous for me and she is still worried that I don't get enough sleep.

She said I needed to slow down. I said that I find it hard to say 'no' when I know that if I don't sign up to something, somebody equally as busy as me will have to do it instead. I think that's a common stumbling block for people and is probably what keeps community groups and voluntary organisations going.

Jane looked me in the eye and said that I wouldn't be any use to anyone if I got cancer again. I pondered on the prospect of PTA groups in heaven, and found I was bound to agree. She said that I had to make my decisions in a vacuum, that I had to look at any request for help against the backdrop of my week and assess whether I could agree to it or not. She said that everybody needed to do that. And if none of us had the time to do it, well, the job wouldn't get done. And in that case, maybe it wasn't so important after all.

That was new to me. I'd never made decisions of this nature with my time at the top of the decision making tree before. It was much more about whether I was best placed to do something. Take a car load to a netball tournament? Pick me! I work from home so could slip out and make up the hours later – even if it was at midnight. Help with reading at school? Yes, of course, because they needed somebody. And reading is the bedrock of everything, isn't it?

And availability of time isn't the whole picture, because working with others and helping other people often makes us feel happy and that what we're doing is worthwhile. To take that away might bring more time but with it less contentment and more stress. Jane, calm, demure, oh so caring and yet sleeping eight hours a night, said that was true, but that we were only talking about the odd request here, not shunning all our commitments in life.

I'm glad I've helped a little in the past. We all need to do our bit, don't we? And there are many people out there doing much more than I ever did. But moving forward, if I was to make up for my previous early morning bonus working hours, these days assigned to sleep, I needed to change my mindset.

On the back of my conversations with Jane I have made a few decisions regarding my time, including the decision to stop some voluntary work. And I do feel guilty. It's hard to change the mindset of a lifetime. but it's just the odd commitment and I can always pick it up again later.

And you know, nobody minds, people understand. Never have people been more sympathetic about my need to sleep. I would even go so far as to say that people are more sympathetic to a desire to make life-changing decisions in our lives when we've just had a life-changing illness. If this applies to you then perhaps now is the time to make bold choices because there will never be an easier time to have them accepted.

And if you're a friend or relative looking after someone with cancer, do it now, too. If anyone has a problem with that, smile and do it anyway! Bucket lists are great but we shouldn't have to wait for illness before we start them.

To reconstruct or not to reconstruct

The decision whether to undergo reconstructive surgery is an enormous topic for breast cancer patients and often involves a deeply personal and complicated decision process.

I wanted to talk about it here because my experience would have been different if I'd known what I know now before I had my first mastectomy operation. I certainly would have requested more information and perhaps asked if there was the possibility of a different surgeon to perform the mastectomy. Not, I hasten to add, because mine wasn't perfectly competent in mastectomy operations, but because he didn't do reconstructive surgery and therefore didn't have half an eye on reconstruction later. Knowing what I know now, I should have asked about 'skin sparing' operations and the option to have an 'expander' fitted. If either had been appropriate for me during the mastectomy, it would have given me more options later.

Hospitals pool knowledge to achieve 'best practice' across the NHS, but preferred practice does, nonetheless, differ between hospital trusts. Harrogate hospital, where I received all of my treatment apart from the radiotherapy, 'advised against' having immediate reconstruction following a mastectomy if there was any possibility of needing chemotherapy or radiotherapy. Adding reconstruction into the mastectomy equation, it was explained to me, was a 'much bigger job', which left the patient more prone to infection and other complications. The wound would have to be fully healed before commencing chemo because nobody wants a vulnerable new wound when the body's defences, its white blood cells, are being challenged.

They couldn't risk a wait for the start of my chemo regime so I had a choice of mastectomy followed by chemo or chemo followed by mastectomy, reconstruction only ever being offered at the end of my active treatment. The BCN said that a delayed reconstruction was generally considered to be a good thing as it gave people time to consider the options before making their choice. She had a point. When I was told I needed a mastectomy, about twenty seconds after finding out I had cancer and the infamous, 'It's much worse than we thought,' moment, I remember the 'mastectomy' word barely touched my head, sort of glancing over the top instead. My brain was the Spaghetti Junction in a fog with a sprinkling of Valium. You need to remove my breast, you say? Absolutely! Who needs boobs? Take the other one, too, if you wouldn't mind, and if you'd like a few fingers and toes for good measure, have them with my blessing. All I ask is that you cure me but oh, just leave my heart and brain would you?

Even then, shocked and not really in my body, but hovering above looking down on that poor soul in the room with her stunned husband beside her, having just found out she had cancer, I vaguely remember thinking that if I survived, I might not always think like that.

And I don't.

Reconstruction is a big deal. It's a different undertaking to cosmetic breast surgery which deals with existing, healthy breast tissue. Generally reconstruction is lengthy surgery and often involves more than one operation, each requiring weeks of recovery. It also carries with it a significant failure and complication risk. I don't want to scare you, I just wish I'd entered into the decision making process knowing what reconstruction is about, rather than thinking it involved little more than attaching a piece of silicone in place of the missing breast.

Make sure you know your choices. There are several different types of reconstruction available using either artificial implants or tissue from elsewhere in the body. Not all methods of reconstruction are right for all people and some options need preparation at the time of your mastectomy, even if reconstruction isn't to be considered until months after the end of your active treatment. Your BMI and natural shape ('apples' have more natural tissue options than 'pears'), size of breast, personal taste, work commitments, attitude to surgery and whether you underwent radiotherapy will all play a part in your decision. There's a wealth of information online about the different options, lots of booklets and leaflets available through your hospital and the Macmillan charity, and your BCN will happily arrange an appointment with a consultant surgeon to discuss your options.

My surgeon and oncologist understand both my reservations

yet desire for reconstructive surgery, but I have heard of some surgeons being baffled by a decision not to go for reconstruction. Part of me sees this as a comfort – the operation is clearly not considered a risky undertaking – but the other part of me thinks that all surgery has its risks. I totally understand why people wouldn't want to put themselves or their family through any further 'elective' surgery. My advice is to be kind to yourself. Give yourself time to decide. Remember this is your body, your time, your future. The decision is yours to make and it is a personal one. Due to my body shape, no skin sparing or expander implant at the time of mastectomy, and skin which didn't take kindly to radiotherapy, there are not many options open to me. I also said that you couldn't pay me to have anything other than an essential operation after the infamous artery spurt. But that's my head. In my heart, I still haven't made up my mind.

The good thing is that there is no deadline for reconstruction on the NHS. So there's no hurry to make a decision. If your skin has been affected by radiotherapy, it's likely you'd be encouraged to wait for at least six months, if not a good couple of years after surgery, anyway.

There is a third way which again, has some surgeons baffled and others very supportive, and that is the 'flat' option. Some people opting out of reconstruction would prefer to have the other breast removed as well. The remaining breast, particularly if it's large, lacks symmetry, can cause back ache and of course, always carries the risk of contracting cancer. However, I should point out here that we are constantly reassured that a woman who has had breast cancer in one breast (without genetic links), is only marginally more likely than a woman who hasn't had breast cancer, to contract cancer in the other. Nonetheless, any increased risk doesn't sit easily with someone who has had cancer and the opportunity to take away this fear and have symmetry again, can be very appealing.

Personally, I think if we happily offer patients reconstructive surgery, then we should also offer the less complicated operation to remove the second breast. Not all hospitals see it this way, however, and the general practice is that a patient requesting the 'flat' operation is required to meet with a psychiatrist to check that they are of sound mind. I am all for this on one level, these are enormous decisions and I'd welcome an expert to endorse any choice I make. But I find it odd that a person opting for reconstruction isn't required to have a similar meeting with a psychiatrist. It's as if the decision to have such large scale surgery is the sane one. I have not gone for the flat option but know people who have and who are very happy with their choice. They'd like the choice to be available to all and that's something I support. If you'd be interested in learning more about this option or find you decide against reconstruction, a supportive group of like-minded souls can be found here –
http://www.flatfriends.org.uk/

A Little Less Squished

Roll over Dickens and Tolstoy.

A Squash and a Squeeze by Julia Donaldson, the favourite rhyming book of my then toddler, has had such an impact on my life. I'm not sure how much of the moral my youngest took in at the time – that everything in life is relative and happiness lies in appreciating what you have –but she certainly went to sleep with a smile after numerous renditions of, 'Glory me! It was tiny for two and it's titchy for three'.

Little did I know that I'd still be quoting *A Squash and a Squeeze* long after the screams of, 'Take in my hen? What a curious plan,' had turned to the killing fields of the Hunger Games.

In *A Squash and a Squeeze*, the wise old man asks the farmer's wife to trust in his philosophy. Her poky house is getting her down and she doesn't have room to 'swing a cat', let alone her farm animals of assorted sizes, which the wise man asks her to add one by one into her already straining abode. It's only when he directs her to remove them that she realises quite what she had before.

2014 has been a bit of a squash and a squeeze for me and none more so than the summer holidays, rammed with radiotherapy appointments at the expense of work and being with (and transporting) my teenage children. Where the old lady filled her house one by one with extra animals varying in size from a hen to a cow, my 2014 was filled with treatments for cancer. But as in the book, it's all relative; I am one of the lucky ones. That doesn't mean I haven't lamented the lack of time.

Throw in chemo! the oncologist said.
I can't I cried. I teach, I edit, I write
I work for my husband (badly), have a small business
(which suddenly seems humongously large)
and short stories and a novel I'm trying to type.
And I want to ride my bike.
I can't take on chemo, my life is a squash and a squeeze.

But in the chemo went.

Take out a week every three to recuperate
And add in Herceptin every three weeks for a year
And radiotherapy.
Oh! don't shed a tear, after 15 sessions you'll be out of here.
And then add in Tamoxifen for the next nine years and one
It's only a pill, with any luck, it won't make you ill.

And then I blinked and it was September. The big cow had stopped dancing on the dining room table. I locked the door soundly behind it. Goodbye chemo, farewell, I hope. Radiotherapy has been winched out of the top window. In the kitchen there are still a few hens pecking at my feet; a reminder that this cancer journey still rolls on but I can manage perfectly well even with a constant tickle at my toes.

So sympathetic, professional and advanced has been my treatment that although I breathe in the less cluttered air with relish, there is a part of me which hasn't disliked the squash and a squeeze of the last nine months. I've found it interesting, supportive, friendly and hopeful. I'd have gladly done without it, but without the brilliance of the medical profession and the incredible love and support of those around me, the path life has forced me down would have been much less bearable.

And let's face it; I might not have been walking it at all.

My cancer journey isn't over. I can't imagine it ever really coming to an end, although an all–clear after five years is a milestone I wish on every wishbone to meet. Nine months after diagnosis, however, emotionally and practically, I'm feeling a little less squished.

The new normal

Breast cancer treatment is likely to induce a premature menopause. Yep, I nearly fell off my chair when I heard that one. And I'm afraid there is no warning, no warm up, and no gentle slide in. No, those hormones are switched off in an instant by chemo and kept that way by Tamoxifen and similar drugs (if your cancer is hormone receptive). And your body doesn't care for it one little bit.

Of all the potential side-effects of cancer treatment, somehow the prospect, and I'm afraid, also the reality of a premature menopause depressed me the most. Cancer was going to make me old before my time and that wasn't fair because I'd planned to hit the ground running and catch up exactly where I'd left off just as soon as the active treatments had finished. I can't pretend I'm happy about the situation even now but I am coming to terms with it. The good news is that I haven't picked up my zimmer frame just yet.

I've exchanged Chemo Brain for Tamoxifen Confusion mixed in nicely with Menopausal Madness. Pre-chemo and Tamoxifen, I pretty much had a handle on things. I knew where each of my three other family members were at any given time, even if they didn't. The, Mum! I can't find... was met with, If I have to look and find it within ten seconds, you owe me 10p. And I knew I'd be quids in. Mum, they said, are my skinny jeans clean? They are, I'd say, washed this morning, on the airer now, another three hours twenty minutes to go. That's your black ones, the blue ones with the ripped knees are in the machine as we speak and the green ones are waiting to be ironed. Menopausal Madness? Well, the washing goddess crown has well and truly slipped down over my eyes. Oh, have you got some skinny jeans? I say. That's nice.

And don't even get me started on work. Thank the lord for my Filofax. Forget electronic devices, I need my Filofax laid open beside me at all times so that I can check whether I've responded to the email I read a moment before, to remind myself what I've already done and what I need to do next. Life was certainly simpler back when I could keep all this stuff in my head. But it isn't anything that diligent note and diary keeping can't handle, even if it is a little tedious and frustrating.

What else? Well, I'm osteopenic, which means my bones aren't as strong as they could be, but I don't yet have full blown osteoporosis. That means more drugs and a prayer or two that my bones won't start cracking. Thankfully I have a running addiction on my side, because weight bearing sports are your best line of defence against thinning bones, which come to all women if they live long enough. And hey, it gives me a good excuse to prioritise running over cleaning. The impact on my femininity, the re-distribution of fat stores – i.e. fat ass – a lack of energy, joint ache and the hot sweats which make me look like an embarrassed teenager by day and wake me up in a pool of sweat at night, all seem to come as a package with this early menopause lark. I can't pretend I like it.

The difference between a chemo and Tamoxifen induced premature menopause and the onset of the natural menopause, is that the latter is often a more gentle slide in with perimenopausal symptoms first, and the option to take HRT or herbal alternatives later. Obviously, this is not an option for people on Tamoxifen and similar drugs. The oncologist would take a dim view of people putting the oestrogen back which that little box of tablets is doing its utmost to take away. But the good news is that the wonderful cancer calming machine wants to help and there are a few strategies I have tried which have been wonderful.

So, what are these pesky side-effects and what can we do about it?

Warm Flush

Most well documented is the Warm Flush. Warm flush? Warm flush! It makes it sound like something sent to try Jane Austen as she and the female contingent of Mansfield Park subtly fan a little breeze to cool their warm faces. I'm afraid it isn't a Warm Flush but a Hot Sweat and when it comes on at night, it wakes you up, generally in a pool of sweat. Lovely. When it hits you in the day, it starts with a suggestion of heat in the toes, becomes a swell of warmth travelling quickly though the body and culminates in a clammy and glistening pink face. Nice. In public? Keep smiling. You're probably not the only one and my children assure me that my face isn't as puce as it feels.

But, dear body, why oh why? There are a few different theories to explain the warm flush but here's my layman's version. Hormones keep human bodies going. They're the boss pouring just the right amount of oil onto the cogs to make the body go round. In theory, the parts are complete without the hormones sticking their oar in, but the component parts won't glide and chuckle along in harmony without our hormones controlling the system from behind the scenes.

Chemo and Tamoxifen, and related drugs, upset or remove the oestrogen hormone from our bodies. I'm not best of friends with oestrogen because it is likely to have played a part in creating my hormone receptive breast cancer, but generally it's a force for good. After all, we couldn't reproduce without it.

Oestrogen also has a relationship with the hypothalamus which controls temperature. When hormones are balanced and the hypothalamus is working tickety-boo, our temperature fluctuations are kept in check by the hypothalamus. Without its former quota of oestrogen however, the hypothalamus is hampered and starts to behave more like the first BBC Computer than a new Windows PC, and becomes incapable of preventing our temperature from rising.

The effect is compounded at night with pillow-induced hot headedness. Our pillows retain some of the heat naturally emitted from our heads as we sleep, which then begins a perpetual circle: the heat from our head warming the pillow which warms our head which warms our pillow and so the process continues until we've woken every half hour in the night, red hot and perspiring.

1. **Chillow Pillow**

   Welcome: the Chillow Pillow. This is a permanently cold slab upon which daring, brave and very hot souls can lay their head directly. Thankfully, you can also sandwich a Chillow between two pillows for a less extreme chilling method.

   The effects of this little beauty were instant for me. I went from weeks of exhaustingly broken sleep to now barely waking at all. I do think if we can manage to sleep, everything in life is easier.

2. **Water**

   I have always drunk a lot of water so probably can't really comment on this personally. However I have plenty of anecdotes from fellow sufferers to say that drinking copious amounts of water has helped them. And as it's good for so many things, I'd say you have nothing to lose by giving it a go.

3. **Caffeine**

   I've also read a lot about reducing caffeine intake to limit the hot sweats. However, an article in the Mail

Online in April 2015 reported that drinking two coffees a day increased the efficacy of Tamoxifen. The NHS examined the findings, describing them as 'interesting' and 'promising' but currently, inconclusive. It might be worth reading the article however, if you are considering cutting out caffeine altogether – **http://www.nhs.uk/ news/2015/04April/Pages/Coffee-could-make-breast- cancer-drug-tamoxifen-more-effective.aspx**

4. **Alcohol**

Alcohol is high on the list of substances which can increase the incidence of hot flushes. I certainly found a direct link between red wine and the number and severity of my hot sweats. I'd barely take a sip and whoosh, there went the rush of heat from my toes to my forehead. Interestingly, my other tipples, white wine and Prosecco, don't seem to have the same affect. Red wine also gives me twitchy legs, a phenomenon otherwise confined to pregnancy and the chemo period in my life. As I now have a seven units of alcohol per week limiter fixed in my brain, it makes sense to drink what I like best and what likes me best. Red wine has thus been expelled from my life. There are frequent reports that a glass a day can reduce the risk of heart disease but, and apologies for being such a crashing bore, so can broccoli.

5. **Acupuncture**

I've talked about the therapeutic bonus of acupuncture but it's also used widely to alleviate a number of menopausal symptoms, particularly hot sweats. It worked for me. I had my sessions for free through the wonderful Haven centre, and other similar organisations as well as the cancer centre at your local hospital are likely to offer the service.

6. **Nicotine**

I've never smoked but 'they' say that it can contribute to hot sweats, amongst all the other horrors.

7. **Layers**

You may like this excuse to add to your wardrobe. I love nothing more than a big chunky knit with a fulsome roll-over neck for those frosty wintry days. However, such jumpers are not so agreeable when you're in the throes of a hot sweat. I didn't realise this at first and had a particularly scary claustrophobic moment 'stuck' inside one such jumper at a choir rehearsal. Singing is clearly another of those unlikely pursuits which can raise your temperature. I had to sprint out to the toilets, remove said pullover, fan myself with a paper towel and spot my face and wrists with cold water, before I could replace my pullover and slip back to the arias (OK, I think it was ABBA). That was the last time I wore a jumper all winter, equipping myself instead with layers, particularly cardigans, which would be frequently removed and added. By the way, the menopause can cause 'cold flushes', too. As the incidence of hot flushes has diminished so much these days, I'm looking forward to donning my chunky knits again next winter. Pray for a crisp one for me, would you?

8. Take warm baths or showers

You know, I firmly believe that you have to fit changes to your lifestyle into your, well, lifestyle. I love hot baths and hot showers slightly more than I hate hot flushes. And so I ignore this one. It means I have to sit in the bathroom with the window open in December before I can contemplate going to bed after a hot bath, but for me, this is a price worth paying. I should also say that hot temperatures are to be avoided if you have a risk of lymphoedema.

9. Medication

If none of the above are working, there are some medications primarily used for other ailments such as depression and high blood pressure, for example, which have been shown to alleviate hot flushes. If your symptoms are severe, it might be worth asking your doctor about these.

10. **Cognitive Behavioural Therapy**

You could also ask to be referred for Cognitive Behavioural Therapy (CBT) which changes how we respond to certain stresses and has been shown to have a potential effect on hot flushes as well as other emotional and physical side-effects of cancer.

It appears that the body does find a way of coping with its upset hypothalamus after a while, even if the effect of a premature menopause is generally not reversible, at least not in those over forty at onset. My body is fifteen months down the line, a little bruised and confused by it all, but nonetheless sleeping at night and managing to smile through the pink face episodes, pleased it's still allowed coffee and Prosecco, and happy that for these particular legs, running is not a chore.

Of course nobody needs me to tell them that big changes in our hormones, whether it be in our teens or at specific points in our menstrual cycle, can cause mood swings. And the menopause is well known for producing irritable, forgetful, weepy alter egos of our former placid and fun-loving selves. Sigh. You'd have to ask my family to find out how badly I've been affected...

But help is out there in the shape of medication, nutrition and supplements, behavioural therapies – particularly mindfulness – as well as, here I go again, exercise and fresh air. Please don't suffer in silence.

Tamoxifen

Before I started taking Tamoxifen I hadn't really dwelled on the potential side-effects. I was a little wary as my body never coped well with the pill and boasts an 'impressive' reaction to strong medication. This was the reason my midwife insisted that if I ever found myself in labour again, that I ask for only a quarter of a dose of Pethidine next time. It's also the reason why I continued to have an infusion of Herceptin in hospital rather than a standard dose injection at home. But, slight concerns aside, I was quite excited about starting my five years, now likely to be ten, of Tamoxifen, or a similar post-menopausal version. You know I like to make changes to the body-that-got-cancer and Tamoxifen was certainly one of those.

I took my first tablets when I was on holiday in France and at first thought I'd eaten a dodgy mussel, so bad were the stomach cramps and nausea. My bones ached. Had I over-done it cycling with my husband and brother-in-law, both stronger cyclists than me at the best of times? And when had I got so close to nettles? Oh wait, the nettle rash which had started on my calf was now on my shoulder and now it was on my stomach. Incidentally, the rash coincided with our arrival in the South West of France for the beach part of our holiday so I was looking particularly ravishing with my blotchiness in the 30 degree heat, my bald head in a bandana and a scarf covering my burnt, blistered skin from radiotherapy. Regarding the blistering, I had a slightly different system due to reduced fat around my heart – who knew! – that carried with it a higher risk of skin damage, so please don't think this will necessarily happen to you.

Suddenly it dawned on me that all these ailments could be linked and an hour spent online searching the potential side-effects of Tamoxifen, corroborated that. I rang my oncologist friend (I know, it's a total abuse of our friendship and she's so lovely, she pretends it isn't), who said that if the side-effects were too much, I should stop taking Tamoxifen for a week and then re-introduce it as a smaller dose later. But there was no chance of me doing that. Tamoxifen is a long term treatment and a few missed doses here and there don't dramatically alter its effectiveness. But my brain processes these things differently so I wasn't going to take that risk.

The good news is that the side-effects quickly eased and after nine months, I'm left with a tolerable general queasiness, slightly achy bones and fewer flushes.

Tamoixifen and weight

Forget the millions spent on chemical warfare, tell most women that they will need to take a drug called Tamoxifen which will slow down metabolism, re-distribute fat and, horror of horrors, increase appetite – and then stand back. Tamoxifen is the wonderful drug we love to hate. I try not to be bothered about such trivialities as weight gain. I remind myself how grateful I am that there is an extra agent available to me in medicine's tirade against a return of cancer, which wouldn't be of use to me if my cancer wasn't 'hormone receptive'. I recall that when I found out that I was to take Tamoxifen, I was very relieved indeed. But it would be churlish of me to pretend that I am always totally grown up about its side-effects.

When I heard that the drug would slow down metabolism and increase appetite, I told myself that I would simply have to be more disciplined. I've always had a 'healthy' appetite, piling up my food on my plate, and my weight hasn't really changed since I was 18. That's largely because I much prefer 'healthy food'. I think it's tastier. I don't have a very sweet tooth although I like chocolate and the idea of cakes but I generally find that all cakes taste the same. High fat foods generally make me feel nauseous so I give them a wide-berth, too. I'd always loved my sport and would generally eat to appetite meaning that if I'd just done a four hour bike ride, I'd graze for hours afterwards until I finally sat down to a proper cooked meal. Sitting writing at my desk was different, I'd try to squeeze in a piece of toast before 3pm.

So, pre-Tamoxifen, if I was hungry, I'd eat. If I wasn't, I wouldn't. It was an easy version of the '5:2 Diet'. Some days more, some days less, but no days telling myself that I could eat something else simply because I 'hadn't eaten much today'. In my experience, dieting makes you fat and eating to

Fighting Cancer, Living Life

appetite keeps your weight healthy.

Post-Tamoxifen I tried to tell myself that I would have to eat differently. I'd have to be conscious of how much I ate. I'd have to be careful. Other people manage it, why not me?

But the reality is that I find it difficult. The brain is so annoyingly strong and when it's sending messages to your body that you are absolutely starving (even though you've just eaten a week's worth of porridge in one sitting and it's barely 10am) and cannot possibly concentrate on anything until some calories have gone in, it's really hard to ignore. We try not to be vain, and are so thankful for still being around to be bothered, but anybody of normal BMI or above who says they are happy to put on weight, I suspect isn't being entirely truthful.

I did put on weight when I first started with Tamoxifen. I became much more of a snacker, and those brain messages contrived to win much of the time. I didn't like it. My clothes didn't fit like before and I was loathe to go out and buy anything in the size above.

Cancer was not going to beat me this far down the line.

I realised that if I was going to actually be able to concentrate and do any work at all with the voice in my head screaming constantly that if I didn't eat now I would pass out, I would have to pacify Voracious Appetite (VA) with innocuous snacks. Nuts aren't exactly low in calories but they are high in nutrition and 'good fats'. There is some thinking that walnuts may help in the anti-cancer fight and so, rather than taking a handful of nuts, I'd take one at a time in the hope that would quash the appetite at least for a few more minutes. There's a bit of a movement against fruit and the sugars in it, currently, but personally I think I need fruit in my life more than I don't, so I would snack on low fat and highly nutritional fruit, in the hope VA would be pacified with that.

The great news is that the effects seem to have calmed down in a few short months. I wonder if my brain has realised that it got it wrong, worked out that it doesn't need more calories when I've already eaten the contents of the cereal cupboard. Maybe my body has adjusted to the new hormonal normal. Maybe I've had to adjust, too. I am more wary about what I eat these days which annoys me. I wrestle with the fact that a drug has changed this for me. But there is no point in being bitter about something designed to give you the best chance of guarding against recurrence or secondaries. And Tamoxifen, or a version of it, is going to be prescribed to me for ten years so it makes sense to get used to it sooner rather than later.

Something to consider

I've noticed, corroborated by others I've met who have been treated at different hospitals around the UK, that the recommendation is to eat heartily to keep your strength and weight up when you're on chemo. Eat anything, they told me, you can lose weight after treatment.

The trouble with chemo is that it affects your taste buds and it's amazing the effect this has on your eating. I remember eating five bowls (sssh! I know) of white sauce one Sunday lunch when I was particularly struggling with the side-effects of chemo: weird taste sensations, mouth ulcers and my chemo cough and sore throat. The Sunday roast just hadn't done it for me, but the white sauce was the first thing I'd eaten in weeks which tasted exactly as it should so I only stopped eating when it ran out. I didn't feel guilty at all. I felt great. So I do understand that life is different when you're on chemo and you have to do whatever gets you through. But you'll probably have days when you feel ok and others when you actually feel good and I would suggest that on those days you try to eat healthily. You will feel better for it if you're filling your body with nutrients and minerals rather than sugar. And the harsh truth is that it is often harder than it might have been to shift weight when you're on hormone treatment so it would be preferable not to put the weight on before you start.

I'm not sure the medical teams will tell you this but that's the word from the coalface.

Different brands

It's easy to forget that Tamoxifen is our friend in all this, standing hand on hips between a potential cancer cell and the oestrogen which bad cells need to do their worst, because it does come with a trolley full of side-effects. My advice would be to try different brands of Tamoxifen. It's widely found that people behave differently with different brands. I know, for example, that the Wockhardt brand is kindest to me and that I must avoid Teva and RelonChem if I want to sleep at night. Other people I know suffer tremendous joint pain with Wockhardt or will trawl around the supermarket chemists with their prescription in hand, only happy when they've located a box of Teva. So, it's worth 'shopping around'. Once you find a brand you like, try to stick with it because changing brands also exaggerates the side-effects. This isn't always easy. Pharmacies have to work to budget like the rest of us and they will, of course, aim to buy the cheapest brand available. This is a quality of life issue though, and a note from my GP to our dispensing pharmacy has helped me to secure my brand of choice, most of the time.

Tamoxifen can make me nauseous but I was advised to try taking it just before bed rather than in the morning and this significantly relieved the symptoms. Taking half of the dose at night and the other half in the morning is also often suggested.

The side-effects of Tamoxifen and the menopause are frustrating but they don't have to take over our lives. I look around me at older women who have clearly come through the other side of the menopause. They aren't all sitting around with perspiring faces, looking glum one minute and shouting at innocent passers-by the next, eschewing food because they feel queasy, or binge eating because their brain demands that they eat.

I leave you with this quote from a friend:

Do you know, one of the unexpected nice things about menopause has been the way in which the women I know have really supported each other, opened up, shared. It's been a huge web of support which sometimes (in my doubtless hormonal state) makes me feel just a little bit emotional.

What do you Say?

What do you say to someone diagnosed with cancer? Of course, everyone reacts and deals with their diagnosis differently so there can be no rights and wrongs – after all, one man's compliment is another woman's smack in the teeth.

But in my own experience, and in listening to other people who have cancer, there are some common statements issued in good faith by caring souls who believe them to be soothing and consoling, which prove to be the opposite. And as it's frequently said that people don't know what to say when they find out their friend, relative or colleague has cancer, I thought I'd pick out a few classic comments where I suggest you proceed with caution.

Please don't have nightmares. Much more than the clangers, we talk about the wonderful love and support which gets us through the tricky times. And I can honestly say that nobody has said anything that's made me cross or any more upset than I currently was – apart from the person who insisted on telling me a statistic about prognosis she'd read, but even that was said in good faith. Compassion, whatever the wording, should never be criticised.

Besides, I'm sure I was guilty of some of these myself...

1. **We could all be run over by a bus**

   Yes, we could, and I appreciate the sentiment. But
   crossing the road is a risk we take; having cancer is
   somewhat forced upon us and when we have it, the
   reality of a premature end is so much more blatant than
   the potential to find ourselves under the wheels of a
   bus. I would also say that if we were particularly worried
   about being run over by a bus, we could take precautions
   to prevent this unfortunate incident such as never
   crossing a road. I, and everyone I know who's been
   touched by cancer, would like to be told the one thing we
   must do to prevent cancer coming back. And we'd all
   do it. Unlike not crossing a road, this hasn't been
   discovered yet.

2. **My friend's brother's sister's cousin had breast cancer
   twice and is fine**

   I understand this one entirely. We all love a success story.
   Surely when someone has cancer, they also want to hear
   success stories, right?

   Sort of.

   But it's a certain kind of success story. Having cancer is
   about having your mortality thrust in front of your face.
   However aware you were of it before, it's just so much
   more immediate now. On diagnosis, I'd suggest there are

two questions that people need answered, hopefully in the affirmative: Can I be cured? and, Can I stop it coming back? With cancer, one of the hardest things to believe is if you're lucky enough to survive the first time, that your body won't get it wrong the next time. When those rogue cancer cells called, your body was found wanting. What logic says your defences will perform better next time? A lot of logic, actually. There's plenty of research and a wealth of stats to show that your body won't get caught out again, and drugs such as Tamoxifen and Herceptin also help your body change its attitude. But whatever the scientists tell us, it takes time to trust your body again after cancer. If you have breast cancer and have had one breast removed, it's really hard to rationalise that you're not going to get cancer in the other one. And next time it might be harder to detect. It might have spread further. It might be more difficult to cure. And even if all the answers were positive, who would relish the idea of another round of treatments?

So, I suggest proceeding with caution in the choice of success stories. Those where people have survived multiple incidences of cancer are another resounding endorsement that recurrence happens. And that isn't something that somebody who's currently dealing with a primary cancer, wants to think about.

3. **I've just read an article that if you snort three pieces of seaweed (freshly picked that morning from anywhere along the beach between Seahouses and Alnwick on the north coast) on the hour, every hour, they said it could reduce the risk of cancer**

    I'm all for well-researched information which has scientific backing. Trust me, I'm as keen as anyone to discover a food source which will give me that piece of mind. But one person's chance hearing can be another person's twenty-four hours of research and if you magnify that by all the good folk who've heard a rumour, all of a sudden you're wading through a confusion of unsubstantiated research where it might have been much better for your health to relax and read a book. The most helpful suggestions are from those who hear something, carry out the research and only pass on the findings when they've done the work for you. Some people have done this for me and I really appreciate it.

4. **We're all going to die anyway**

    Yes, we are. However, most of us hope that if we do our best to treat our body with respect, we'll live beyond retirement. It isn't something I take for granted but it is a hope. So yes, we will all die one day but when you've just been diagnosed with cancer at 45, your biggest fear is that the day could be forty years earlier than it might have been.

5. **What's the prognosis?**

   No. Just no. Nobody has asked me this but I was staggered to hear that it was quite a common question and generally from relative strangers. Eeek! I don't think you need me to point out that if somebody hasn't discussed their prognosis, they probably don't want to talk about it. It isn't something you'd forget to mention.

6. **Re chemo aches and groans: at least it means it's working**

   It doesn't mean it's working. It doesn't mean anything significant and the inaccuracy of this upsets some people.

7. **Re pending chemo: does it make it easier now you know what to expect?**

   I think this might be acute paranoia on my part but it feels like the awfulness of chemo is belittled with this question. It's as if, had you'd been stronger or braver rather than fearful for previous doses, the experience wouldn't have been as bad. In truth, knowing what's coming is more likely to make it worse.

8. **You look great**

   Usually said when you don't and /or you feel terrible. This offends some people but not me, I LOVE this one, you can tell me as many times as you like!

A little more about stats

Stats go hand in hand with cancer treatment and diagnosis like flies and a Venus Fly Trap.

Because every cancer behaves slightly differently in our unique bodies and environment, the medical experts can't categorically know which bodies will beat cancer and which ones won't. Instead they have to work on likelihood. They produce evidence based stats which tell us how many people with a similar combination of factors (size of tumour, grade and spread) survive two years, five years and sometimes ten years post diagnosis. Of course, it would be better if they could produce a crystal ball to tell us whether we're going to live or die, but of course, cancer isn't that kind of disease.

I've noticed that carers of people with cancer are often interested in stats. And they'll rummage through a myriad of scenarios on-line to find the number they want to see. To them, a stat in excess of 50% positivity, perhaps even less so, might be encouraging. After all, the odds are in their loved one's favour.

In my experience however, those people with cancer, the ones who 'already are the stat', aren't so keen to hear them. Even if 90% of people are expected to survive with no recurrence or secondaries, why wouldn't you be in the 'other' 10%? When you were already the 1:8 who will develop breast cancer at some time in their lives, why wouldn't you be, 'the one' again?

It isn't a case of 'Why me?' but 'Why not me?' I was deemed a more 'unusual' stat because I had no risk factors – although in reality, I've found that my situation isn't that unusual at all. Plenty of young people who've never smoked or drunk excessively, generally eat healthily, like their sport and have no family history of cancer, contract cancer. Nonetheless, it's hard to believe that if my body could defy the odds and get cancer in the first place, that it wouldn't go down that route again.

Thus, the only statistic I would be interested in reading would be of a 100% certainty of no recurrence or secondaries, and as nobody, not even those apparently healthy and certainly not having had a brush with cancer, is said to have a 100% chance of surviving the next ten years, that isn't going to happen. For that reason I steer well clear of statistics and prefer to rely on my head to have a stiff word with myself. I preach the, 'perfect storm' theory. Lots of things, in fact all the body's natural cancer defences, have to fail simultaneously for cancer to form. Bad cells have a go constantly, but most of the time the body is way too clever with far too many safety nets for cancer to take hold.

The other difficulty with statistics about survival rates in cancer is that they are often out of date, which presents a far gloomier picture than is the actual truth. Improved treatments, screening and better early detection techniques have had a massive impact on survival rates and prolonging life in recent years.

Somebody I know impressed a stat upon me because she just couldn't believe I wouldn't be cheered by it. I spoke over the top of her, asking her not to talk about stats, and she told me anyway because she thought that I would appreciate it once I knew. It was done in good faith but I was absolutely crestfallen. By only using recognised sites on the internet, ones that I knew purposely hid their stats away behind tabs so that they couldn't be happened upon by chance, I'd managed to totally stay away from them. But she caught me off guard. I tried to put the stat to the back of my mind but I can't forget it. Even though my rational self knows that the stat is very promising, I wish I didn't know it.

For all these reasons, may I suggest caution if you're feeling inclined to console a friend or relative with what seems an overwhelmingly positive stat to you? Ask them if they're interested in stats before you tell them. Most people I know have a strong view on this. This person was well-meaning but her good intentions took me to a place I didn't want to go.

What do you do?

In my last post I talked about those well-meaning throwaway comments made to people with cancer which might have less than the desired effect. I found it a tricky post to write as uppermost in my mind was the fact that nobody wishes to offend and everybody means to say the right thing. With one man's compliment being another women's slap in the face, it's a minefield for those without privileged entry into a cancer sufferer's chaotic mind. Nonetheless, I hope the post was useful. Your responses were, as ever, thoughtful and touching.

I'm happy to say that I'm back in my comfort zone with this post. It was inspired by the lovely Chriss Green, prolific sharer of my blog for which I'm supremely grateful, who suggested I list things people have said which hit a good spot.

I started scribbling immediately but quickly realised that it was the things people DID rather than what they said, which stuck more in my mind. So, instead of words, I've listed some of the bountiful gifts and good deeds people have bestowed upon me over the past ten months. This isn't a definitive list of how to empty your money box or eat up your already hard-pressed time when you find out someone close to you is suffering, and it won't be for everyone. But I hope my experience might offer a few nuggets of usefulness.

And at least I get the chance to say thank you :)

1. **Meals on Wheels**

   People would ask me to let them know what help I
   needed. They truly wanted to help – but it feels wrong
   to ask somebody with a job, various children, a dog,
   family taxi service and clean house to manage, to run
   around for me when I'm confined to the sofa.

   This doesn't mean that help wasn't gratefully received –
   even getting dressed was a bit of an effort on my worst
   treatment days – and so to open my door on several
   mornings to find a meal for four requiring only a re-heat
   and transportation to the table, was wonderful. My Meals
   on Wheels deliveries made me smile and I'd just like to
   say a public thank you here, as well as an apology for not
   always returning the Tupperware in a timely fashion.

2. **Picking my children up from clubs and feeding them**

   Thank you.

3. **Picking me up from home and taking me for a coffee**

   (and appointments) Thank you.

4. **Supermarket delights**

   With special thanks to the Marks and Spencer Dine-in
   initiative.

5. **Bags of healthy food, home-made chocolate brownies, cakes and bought cakes (I'm not choosy)**

    Thank you.

6. **Loans of DVDs and books**

    Again, thank you.

7. **Messages**

    Personally, I'm not a great fan of speaking on the phone. I blame my poor hearing which makes the process excruciatingly painful for all parties involved. But I had some sleepless nights and painful days through chemo and receiving texts out of the blue saying simply that I was in people's thoughts, was a great tonic. With my treatment induced lethargy however, responding could take chunks out of my day so I hope you'll accept my apology for the tardy replies.

8. **Cards**

    As above. I have kept them all :)

9. **Gifts**

    This may sound terribly materialistic but to know that someone is thinking of you when they go shopping (and I know that often presents came after much research and probing of shop staff's knowledge) touched my heart.

Most practical gift? There were so many! Warm items of clothing went down well – I wore my fluffy pink angora wool socks constantly as well as my Bamboo Chic Lite cardigan. It isn't particularly that treatments make you cold, it's just that our house is Baltic if you aren't running up and down the stairs every second minute.

Most used item? Probably my Anastasia Beverly Hills eyebrow kit. People expressed their delight that I'd held onto my eyebrows. I hadn't ;) Luxury hand and body creams were also a great buy as cancer treatments really dry out the skin. I was lucky enough to be given lots of luscious products I wouldn't normally afford which I'm still using now.

Most tear-inducing? My four-leaf clover bracelet, four-leaf clover necklace (there's a theme here), message and pocket sized hearts. And don't get me started on the handmade ring given to me shortly after the wedding of one of my closest friends, which I couldn't attend due to an incredibly poorly timed third operation.

10. **Home visits?**

I learnt something about myself during chemo: I don't like to see people when I'm ill. I prefer to lick my wounds on my own, cushioned by my home. And then when I'm recovered, that's when I like to see people. Of course, one person's nightmare is another's delight so it's probably worth asking the question.

11. **Showing you know**

Everybody wants the cancer to be treated and consigned to the past post haste. Having treatments behind you is wonderful but the fear that the cancer will return is massive. Mentally, I've needed my friends and family more post treatment than during it. While you're to-ing and fro-ing to hospital for the potpourri of chemicals and radiation assigned to you, you're invincible. The brilliance of modern science and your medical team are all over this little cancer blighter. Pah! Those piffling little cancer cells won't have a chance against drugs which make your hair fall out and turn your bones to putty.

But when treatment ends and it's you, your body and a measly little pill fighting the good fight, staying mentally strong enough to banish the fear to the back of your mind can be tough, particularly when every drug-induced side-effect or contact with bugs feels incontrovertibly like the return of cancer. Those of us who have beaten cancer or who are in remission are the lucky ones and I never forget that, but sometimes the dark thoughts can be over-powering and it's easy to feel a little alone at this post-treatment time.

We're all so busy and I personally find that as soon

Fighting Cancer, Living Life

as one person I know edges out of a crisis situation, another moves in. But *showing you know* doesn't have to be time-consuming. A word or a hug to remind your friend that you know the shadow of cancer is still pretty overwhelming, or that the side-effects of drugs can be depressing, might be all your friend needs to help them get on with the business of living.

12. **Timing**

Anyone who's had a baby will know that when your new-born is tiny and cute and sleeping a lot, everybody comes to visit. Then the visits stop and you're left with the magnitude of looking after this new little person who is sleeping less, feeding more and creating mountains of washing. Right now is when you could really do with someone holding the baby while you put the tea on.

Cancer is a little bit like that. Lots of people visit at the beginning and it's a very human, touching reaction. But if you're well before treatment starts, this period can be very busy. The same pending-birth-nesting need kicks in and suddenly having clean bed linen, every item of school uniform washed and neatly pressed, full cupboards, full freezer and a sparkling toilet ready before your operation becomes monumentally important. And then there's the children's schedule to organise for the three weeks post-op when you won't be driving – the *cancer will not make them miss out on any of their activities* mantra beating inside your head – supper to arrange because you won't be entertaining for a while, and work to finish for previously made deadlines set smack in the middle of a dose of morphine.

So, I'd like to suggest you take the pressure off yourself. Visits are lovely but don't feel guilty if you can't rush around the moment you find out – sending a message and arranging to meet once your friend is out of hospital might actually be more relaxing and helpful for both.

So, that's my list. Can you add any top tips? I love to read your comments. By the way, did I say thank you enough? This wasn't a year I'd choose, but nonetheless I look back upon it with a smile. I've seen lots more of my friends and family than I normally would and who could possibly complain about that?

The Fear

I am not immune to The Fear, unfortunately. I had hoped I might be. Forget piano certificates, gymnastics badges and swimming awards – actually, scrap the swimming awards, I failed the level below my Bronze Survival and had to do the launch of shame from the pool after only the first discipline. I should add that I'd told my teacher I couldn't tread water but she didn't believe me – never do I feel more proud than when hospital staff praise my apparent bravery, my 'high pain threshold'.

I like to test it from time to time, with the odd break of a foot or knee, or the smashing of too many bones in my forearm and wrist, or a chance spurting artery following a fairly routine operation. How's the pain? the nurse asked, as the blood spewed so fast into my chest cavity that, mercifully, the vessels carrying blood from the miscreant area couldn't cope and thus blocked, saving my life (thank you blood vessels) – but oh, at a painful price.

Out of how many? I asked, or rather, wheezed. 10, she said. It's 10, I answered. It couldn't have got any worse than it was and I had to wait three desperately long hours until I could have any form of pain relief. The 'ten' conversation was useful however, as it meant that as the big hand struck 7.05am, the nurse was there, at my side, pouring in the first dose of morphine which she'd set up a few minutes before.

Is this a good point to mention my love for nurses everywhere?

So, with this so-called high pain threshold I'd hoped I'd have nerves of steel and The Fear wouldn't consume me.

And it doesn't consume me. But it does visit often.

Provided The Fear proves unfounded, the further away from initial cancer diagnosis you can step, the more it retreats, I'm told. But for the moment, The Fear of recurrence of cancer is loud; concert pitch on occasion. And although I stuff my fists into my ears, shake my head to disperse the debilitating thoughts, fill my life with family, friends, chocolate and busyness, The Fear is sometimes just too powerful.

My hearing has always been my bug bear. I wear hearing aids. They are wonderful. My tiny friends discretely do their job and I can go about my daily life barely affected, save for the odd mishear, just to keep my interlocutors amused. My hearing is going through a bad phase. I'm constantly reaching for the remote control to turn up the volume of my aids only to realise it's already on maximum. BC – before cancer – I'd have said that my ears must be blocked (I have tiny ear canals, they're easily blocked). BC, my hearing would have sorted itself. Post-cancer, when I can't hear well, I fear I have a brain tumour. The most likely cause is actually a side-effect of

Tamoxifen, the hateful drug we truly love because it may be keeping us alive.

Last week I felt sick and wondered if the cancer had gone to my stomach. In reality, it was simply that-type-of-cold. I could go on.

It's The Fear of those cancer cells dodging the medication, laughing in the face of the operations and lodging themselves into a new area of the body, one not being routinely checked. We tell ourselves that the medication is advanced, clever and designed exactly to deal with the evil little blighters but The Fear reminds us that they are clever, too.

It can be paralysing when The Fear muscles its way into our lives, lodging itself into our psyche and much as we try to ignore it, keeps beating us mercilessly.

But I will not be beaten.

I will not let The Fear win. I ring my doctor. I apologise for my post-cancer paranoid hypochondria and she understands. They all understand. That's the lovely truth of the Cancer World. They expect it. They expect those of us who are lucky enough to have survived and feel guilty that we let The Fear strike when we should be shouting hallelujah for our fortune, to be sitting in their surgeries. And they don't mind; they really don't mind and that does make us feel better.

And each time The Fear comes knocking and the door is answered with a reassurance that all is well, each time that The Fear proves unfounded, then another chip is shaved from the lump lodged in my consciousness, another stone ricochets off the side of Goliath's head. The Fear gradually gets pushed a little closer to the back of my mind and normality is dragged a little closer to the front.

I do not feel the same as I did BC. I do feel a little isolated fighting what sometimes feels like an inevitable recurrence, especially now that the heavies of operations, chemo and radiotherapy have done their bit and the only remaining super power, Herceptin, is drawing to a close. I have two more before I finish my year of dosages. I shan't miss the time out of my Tuesday or the water retention (or, Herceptin Bum) and general grogginess which follows for a few days, but I shall miss the reassurance and friendliness of the nurses and the partial piece of mind this powerful drug gives, when it's just me and Tamoxifen fighting the good fight. The Fear will keep attacking me but I will win eventually, because I will not let it affect my here and now. It's madness, isn't it, to waste the glorious present worrying about the unknown future?

Madness yes, human also, but helpful...not at all.

Beyond the fear

I can't say my trip to Cancerville is completely behind me, nor ever will be. People say your life will be forever changed by cancer and it's true. When the treatments end, our new post-cancer life really begins. It's a life sprinkled with hospital appointments, dark thoughts and irrational fears.

But it is so much more than that.

My new life isn't better or worse, just different. I'm still living life, savouring the moment, planning a little – although I've never been big on planning for the future, save for a few pennies in the piggy bank. And I'm still here. Grateful. Rejoicing. With every new day more and more of us will survive cancer. We live in fortunate times but there's still room for improvement. Research has changed the outlook for many cancer patients, but until cancer becomes totally curable or diagnosable before a lump is even formed, then more needs to be done. Please support fundraising when you can. And be vigilant with your health.

Don't live in cancer's shadow but don't beat yourself up if some days, the enormity of a diagnosis and its ongoing treatments gets a little too much. There's nothing wrong with taking a breath but then we have to close our mouths and get on with the process of living because cancer or no cancer, our time on this earth is short.

My Cancerversary

Today is my one year cancerversary: twelve months to the day I learned I had cancer.

What do you think I'm going to tell you today? the consultant surgeon asked at 2.30pm a year ago, a nurse by his side. My heart slipped a little closer to my stomach.

During the mammogram and ultra sound tests a week earlier, a couple of comments about the lump (which I'd satisfactorily convinced myself prior to the appointment was the innocuous result of hormones) made me nervous. I asked the radiographer what he was looking for. The mammogram suggests pre-cancer, he said. Pre-cancer, I considered, I like the sound of 'pre'. Yes, he said 'pre' is good.

I left the tests to enjoy Christmas, knowing I'd be returning on the 27th December for the results. Then they'd tell me whether I had no cancer or pre-cancer. Or so I thought.

I'd learnt about pre-cancer over the festive period. I didn't go near the internet – am way too cautious to trust my sanity to Mr Google – but instead consulted with my wonderful friend who, rather fortuitously for me, happens to be an oncologist in breast cancer. Pre-cancer wasn't to be taken lightly, I was told. Dependent on the extent of these cells at the first abnormal stage, a mastectomy might be necessary, together with hormone therapy, perhaps, even a dose or two of radiotherapy.

But no chemo and, crucially, no risk of death at this pre-cancerous stage. If there's a sentence containing 'cancer' as well as, 'no risk of death', it's hard to feel anything but relief.

I looked at the surgeon and the nurse and I think I smiled. It was OK, I'd prepared for this and the way he'd phrased the question made me certain. You're going to tell me I have pre-cancer, I finally answered. The surgeon and the nurse continued their gaze, not even a twitch from either of them until the surgeon said, I'm afraid it's much worse than that.

And thus I trot towards 2015 with three operations, chemotherapy and radiotherapy behind me and with much more optimism about the future than I had last New Year's Eve. Nonetheless, I'm celebrating my cancerversary small; just poking a superstitious toe into the festivities. No parties this year, just gratitude for the brilliance of modern medicine and for the love which has helped me step over the pebbles. Some people have to deal with cancer and other crises on their own and I can't begin to imagine how hard that must be. Being with my family around the gold star-bedecked table, clutching a tiddlywink cracker, brought me to tears this Christmas, and not just because I burnt the pigs in blankets. I'm lucky to be here and my cancerversary is a time to give thanks for that.

Next year I hope to celebrate two years clear, then three and four and onto five. Five years is a milestone I pray to reach and a significant goal in the life of Grade 3 breast cancer. That's when we can really believe it's finished: every last stray cell gone, no new little blighters gaining strength and preparing to strike. December 27th 2018 is going to be one heck of a party.

Meanwhile, I shall keep thanking my lucky stars for no signs of recurrence or secondaries. I shall keep checking. You must too, because early detection is your biggest weapon against cancer. Do it on the same day every month and then you won't forget. And boys, no sniggering at the back, you know you have to check yourself too, right?

And most of all I shall keep having fun because none of us know where our life is headed. In the inimitable words of the Cold Feet opening credits: Life's a journey, travel it well.

Cancerversary and time

You've looked forward to this moment, ticked off the chemo sessions and counted down the days, but don't be surprised if you aren't rejoicing when you step out of hospital moments after receiving your final chemo, or even two to three weeks later when the side-effects of your final dose have worn off. Not that it isn't a relief knowing that you don't have to go back and do the chemo cycle all over again. It's just that for me, another emotion was much more powerful: The Fear.

Nurses assured me it is very common to feel flat, emotionally drained and, most of all, scared when active treatment finishes. It's made worse by the pressure we put upon ourselves because we think we should feel wonderful. I didn't feel wonderful. I felt very exposed. Without chemo and radiotherapy in my armour, I, me, Jackie Buxton, seemed a tremendously insipid force as the first line of defence against any resistant stray cancer cells or indeed, new ones.

On another level I felt guilty for not rejoicing: this was the end of my active treatment to rid me of cancer. Other people weren't so lucky.

When I looked in the mirror and saw my bald face and head, I hated looking so poorly when really, I felt quite fit. And I felt guilty for worrying about my appearance when, well, you don't need me to spell it out. Contrary to this being a problem however, a kind nurse said that she would be worried if I wasn't bothered about my appearance, that not caring was a flag in the diagnosis of depression. In fact, I should be relieved to feel glumness.

So I embraced my disdain for my appearance.

I also discussed my post treatment angst with my oncologist who said something which resonated with me. He said that we have to learn to trust our body again and that it takes time. I have learnt that there is no substitute for time and have watched myself through the process of re-gaining trust, with Fear slipping a little further back in my consciousness. And now? I don't think of cancer every minute, or even every hour, but I do think about it several times a day, and more if I have a niggle, because every pain I feel or illness that intrudes into my life irrefutably points to cancer. What else could it be?

Time has helped but there is still some way to go.

Getting cancer is a perfect storm. It takes so much more than a rogue, deformed cell to cause a tumour. Mistakes have to be made many times in the powerhouse of the body for that rogue cell to survive, mutate and recreate. Many a dodgy cell has been rejected post-haste from the body without us ever knowing. I realised that medical staff tended to view the 'perfect storm' as a comfort. What are the chances of it happening again?

Unfortunately I, and other cancer sufferers, fear a different answer to the, 'What are the chances...?' question. We ask ourselves why the storm *wouldn't* happen again when the aspect and weather haven't changed. We are the same body, the same genetics and the same environment as we were before the tumour grew the first time. The evil of cancer liked this environment, this perfect concoction, why wouldn't it like it again?

Time pushes this question further back in our minds. Time helps us to regain trust that lightning doesn't tend to strike twice, even against the same tree. There was something very calming about being told that it would take time to believe this, to begin to trust my body again, that it couldn't be rushed, but that it was inevitable that I would slowly but surely feel more confident and stronger. And that is exactly what is happening. My Cancerversary was almost four months after the end of my radiotherapy sessions which had followed chemo. I raised a quiet glass of bubbly to feeling better. I knew there was some way still to go in my fight against The Fear, but I recognised just how far I'd come since those early days when the end of treatment felt like it might be little more than a holiday in Cancerville.

I'm about to have my last Herceptin infusion after a year of three-weekly doses. I've had no perceptible side-effects and thus the two hour visit to hospital has felt more like an opportunity to have a chat with the nurses again and discuss my hair length. I will miss them.

But I'll also be celebrating. This is another step further away from diagnosis, another treatment completed in which we hope stray cancer cells were annihilated. This is another moment to tell any cells that have designs on mutation, that they can take a running jump.

Did you Watch It?

I've just watched *The C-Word*, the dramatisation of Lisa Lynch's blog, *Alright Tit* (**http://alrighttit.blogspot.co.uk/**) and subsequent book which she wrote about her fight with cancer. Sheridan Smith expertly and touchingly plays the recently married magazine editor who was diagnosed with breast cancer at the desperately young age of 28 and died of its secondary disease five years later. For two years following her original treatment Lisa hoped she was clear of cancer and her life was well and truly back on track.

Then came the line, 'And then the music stopped', which has stayed with me all week.

I was glad I was sitting in the garden, huddled around the fire pit, when it was first aired, as I hadn't decided if I should watch it. I wasn't sure how much the drama could teach me about the experience of breast cancer but knew its potential for sending me into a big dark hole. I'm very protective about what I watch and read. You may know of my aversion to stats, particularly any that touch on that P word: prognosis. It's a word I've come to hate, and I tend to leave it out of sentences and pull a face in its place. Fear of stumbling across a rogue stat is a great incentive to keep me away from the internet and when I'm sent links on breakthroughs and innovative therapies, appreciated as they are, I insist my husband trawls through them for danger zones before I read.

Remember *Brookside*, *TFI Friday*, *Arctic Role*, those frozen mousses in plastic pots, Millennium Eve, *Wham*, *Blind Date*, *When Harry Met Sally*, *The Secret Diary of Adrian Mole* (who is EXACTLY the same age as me, even down to the 3/4), *Bridget Jones Diary* and Le Tour coming to Harrogate? There are certain things in our lifetime which we just have to see, feel, watch or listen to if we want to be fully paid up members of our generation.

I wondered if *The C Word* should be added to this list.

I'll share a secret with you. I was curious that nobody had asked me if I'd watched it. It made me suspicious. I wondered if people thought that perhaps I shouldn't. Or perhaps I might have watched it and been so traumatised that it shouldn't be discussed lest I be propelled down into that dark hole I mentioned. Or perhaps they'd been traumatised themselves. Alas, I am not the only one whose life has been touched by cancer. Whatever the reason, the radio silence was quite a pull towards catch-up TV.

My husband is away and I knew he wouldn't choose to watch it. In real life he is calm. He isn't, 'can be calm,' or, 'is quite calm,' he just IS calm, from his toenails to the hair on his head. When it comes to TV, he is a wimp. *Holby City*? Too much blood. *Call The Midwife*? Why would you want to watch someone scream? *The C Word*? Why would you want to make yourself cry?

It was Saturday night and my eldest was doing eleventh hour replacement pieces for her GCSE Art practical, after her original sculpture snapped only days before its deadline. While I let out a gasp on sight of the photos of the sculpture in too many pieces to count, said daughter, who is her father, just a foot smaller and less hairy, simply shrugged and asked how fast we could get hold of a hardboard mask as she'd had an idea. The other daughter was applying false tan and distracting her GCSE-taking sister into making Dubsmash clips. Do you know about Dubsmash? It's an App. No App ever will make me laugh more than seeing my children performing its videos. If you've watched a programme which has sent you down a dark hole, I promise you Dubsmash is your best chance of clambering back out.

So, with the family absent from the living room, I thought I could sneak a peek without anyone else needing to know.

The problem is that I can't work the television. I never need to switch it on, you see. Like wine and chocolate, TV is a social thing for me, not something I ever do on my own. So I had to ask the Dubsmasher to load *The C Word* for me and thus my cover was rather unglamorously blown. But she wrinkled her nose when she saw the title and slunk back to the Dubsmashing and false-tanning on the bathroom floor, which fortuitously for her requirements (and my carpet), is one of the few places in our house where you can snatch a whiff of Wi-Fi.

Now I was committed.

The C Word didn't have the effect I thought it would. Yes I cried, only perhaps for 90% of it though, and they weren't particularly tears for me. The operations and treatments were all too familiar, as were the feelings and reactions so frankly and eloquently portrayed, but I wouldn't say that *The C Word* brought them all back because they're all still very front of mind. This isn't in a wholly negative way, but in a, 'Phew, that was the year that was,' and, 'Hey, this life without treatments lark is much more fun,' kind of way. Although I would admit that the trials of the side-effects of Tamoxifen also contrive to keep the experience fairly current.

But I did weep for Lisa when she lost her hair. I had forgotten the raw emotion of seeing your identity flushed down the toilet. I'm sure it seems a strange thing to be upset about. Surely it's the least of your worries, right? Wrong! I have a theory. The implications for you and your loved ones of a cancer diagnosis are too big to taste whole, so you have to tackle that enormous universe of uncertainty one atom at a time. Yet your hair is part of a world you do know and understand, and however much you try to be grown up about it, it's way too big a part of your pre-cancer life for you to lose without a great aching lament. It's a deeply sub-conscious thing, but I felt that I couldn't let myself cry about cancer itself. I rarely have which is quite staggering as I'm a bit of a cry baby really. Yet I worried that peeling the lid off the cancer universe might mean I couldn't fit it back on again. Unleash the lava from a volcano and it may never stop flowing. Underneath the despair at holding my hair loose in my hands, I think I knew that my grief for my hair would eventually stop. I think Lisa's writing about this, in a candid and brutal but also wickedly funny way, and Sheridan's portrayal of her vulnerability during this and other stages of treatment captured this brilliantly.

The rest of the tears were for the touching moments with family and friends and in particular with Pete, Lisa's husband. His caring manner and gentle air reminded me of my husband. Yes, I had cancer and yes, I had to undergo more than my fair share of operations and treatments. But I was being looked after and showered with cards and gifts and love and help. My husband, like all those closest to someone with a serious illness or disability, was having to look after me, our children, hold down his job and keep his own sanity – as well as handle his own emotions – pretty much single-handed. My husband, together with my family and friends, are the principal reason why I managed to keep smiling through cancer. People say you are 'strong' and 'brave', but if you're lucky, it's the people around you who really give you strength and courage. And that is what made me cry the most when watching the drama.

The dark hole? I thought *The C Word* might unsettle me for a few hours and then I'd get back on with living. But actually, it had the opposite effect. I found it empowering. The similarities between my and Lisa's lives weren't lost on me: young (-ish in my case), the writing, the blog, the book, even the dressing smart for chemo – chemo power dressing I used to call it. She was even a Virgo!

Much as I ache for Lisa and her family, I pray for the similarities to stop there.

There was nothing Lisa could do when secondaries were silently growing. There's nothing I could do either if it happened but I can do my best to prevent new cancer forming. The C Word was a reminder of my resolve to follow a lifestyle which does its absolute best to repel any further invasion of cancer. As Lisa says, we can't control it, but I can do my best to make my body a fortress of steel against it.

Yes, I sleep much more than I used to but it's easy to let it slide. I mustn't.

My work/ life balance slips into the red zone frequently. I have to address this.

I'm very conscious of how much I drink but that seven unit limit can waver sometimes. I'd love scientists to decide that alcohol would have no ill effect on my health but they won't so I need to get over myself.

And then there's the phone. It's a stress, and I'd been

switching it off at 9pm. Recently it has crept back into my evenings. I've resolved to turn it off again.

And it was a reminder to be bold, proud and alive. Last week I went to the hairdresser and allowed myself to be talked out of having my short hair bleached blonde because it would be too high maintenance. My hairdresser is right of course. But I'd resolved to be bold while my hair grew back into a style which was 'more me', and so tomorrow I'm going back to the hairdresser's. Hang the cost, forget the time, and most of all, sod the commitment. Life, as they say, is too short.

Lisa's story is tragic. People dying of cancer is tragic. People dying before their parents is particularly tragic. But the sad truth is that sometimes illness will win. In the meantime, we should live our lives positively, pack them with experiences while we can, seize the bright side rather than wallowing in regrets, and treat our body with respect so that we give ourselves the best chance of longevity and quality of life. I've always strived to do this and can't really attribute it to Lisa's story. But The C Word was a timely reminder to keep going.

RIP Lisa Lynch and all those who have died too young.

Questions

It amused me that Lisa talked about the fact the cancer was in her right breast as I've always wondered why I found mine in my left. What the devil were my left-sided defences doing when cancer called – snoozing? I have other questions like this:

- Will I have days in the future when I won't think about cancer?
- Do people think I should be 'over it' now, that I should be able to put it to the back of my mind?
- How do I manage to do work I like and still maintain a healthy work-life balance?
- Will *Tea & Chemo* be helpful?
- Will it raise enough money for the charities to make at least a small difference?
- Do people really like my hair or are they just being kind?
- Do people think cancer has changed me? I hope not (unless it's for the better).
- Will my Tamoxifen affected super appetite ever completely wain?
- If I give into it, would there be a point when I'd stop putting on weight or would I just pop one day?
- Will my hair remain dark (before The Grey, at least)?
- Will my children, sisters, mum get breast cancer and will they find it soon enough?
- What is it really like for my husband having a wife who had breast cancer with all its ongoing side-effects?
- Will my children and/ or husband get cancer because we

live in the same environment and eat a very similar diet?

~ Will my eyes ever stop watering?

~ Is my chewing gum habit bad for me?

~ Will there be a point in our lifetimes when there's a vaccine against all cancers?

~ Do I drink too much tea?

~ Will we reach a point when all cancers can be routinely picked up with a blood test in the early stages?

~ How will my children look back on this period of their lives?

Gone Dark Brown

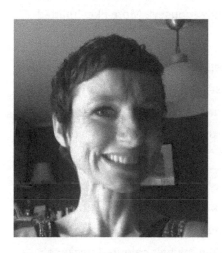

I'm not sure this will be my most profound post ever but I feel an explanation is due for this. I made a promise and I didn't keep it. But I have a reason and I think it's a good one.

Let's go back to a school trip. I forget where we were headed, but sitting near me on the bus was one of those sweet lads who all the girls love but who never has a girlfriend. I remember his name but will protect his identity by calling him Sam. Well, goodness knows how we got onto it but in the middle of a conversation between a group of us fifteen year olds, Sam referred to my hair as, 'mousey'. I was stunned. I'm not sure I'd ever really named the colour of my hair before that but, 'mousey'? Really? Like those little screechy, smelly, runt-of-a-rat type things? Beautiful brunette you hear, blondes have more fun and all that – and hey, who needs brain cells if you're constantly having fun? – but never, 'mesmerising mousey' or, 'mouth-wateringly mousey'. More like, 'matted mousey', perhaps.

Thankfully I managed to keep my horror to myself but it clearly left its mark. I can't say I lost too much sleep over it during the ensuing years but it would be fair to say that if anyone ever asked me what my best feature was, it wouldn't have been the colour of my hair.

So, fast forward, ahem, thirty years to my second lot of baby hair, when it had grown back just enough to potentially push off my wig and cause a scene. I had no choice but to go bare-headed. I decided to have my hair coloured because... well, because I could. The result was a fairly dark brown. I liked it because it made my hair, which you could measure in millimetres, look a fraction longer. That was in December.

Christmas was a memory, January had slipped by and February was as short as ever. March? March was wonderful, we went skiing in Slovakia, just the family, rearranged from a year before when we couldn't go for reasons you know only too well. April? Well, April was seeing the beginnings of a fringe at last so finally I was starting to look less like a rabbit in headlights, or rather, 'Hello! Here comes Jackie's face entering the room'. And then it was May. The dye was incredible. My hair was still dark brown. Not even a whiff of mousey.

In my post I said I was going to go blonde because life was too short. I sat down with the hairdresser and discussed this plan. Why? She asked. Because life's too short, I said. And I want to do something different and the only different I can think of is blonde, dark or red. Red isn't good for me because it makes my skin look like I've just slipped out of intensive care, dark you've already done and thank you, isn't it amazing it's lasted this long and...

When did we dye it dark? she asked. December, I said. December? She laughed. That's not dye, the roots would be this long; and she held out her arms as if she'd just caught a big fish. That's your natural hair colour.

I nearly fell off the pivoting chair. Rather than wondering whether my hair would grow back straight, I should have been asking what colour it would be. The only thought I'd given to hair colour was to brace myself for it coming back grey. That seems to happen a lot. I have no aversion to growing old gracefully (as we all know too well, old is so much better than the alternative) but the drugs had already thrust a *challenging* premature menopause upon me and it would have been nice to have been spared the premature grey, thank you. And I had. Not grey. Not even mousey. But rich brown.

Thank you chemo, that was very kind.

I drifted back from hair Utopia to hear the stylist saying that as my hair was thus now quite dark, the roots would be difficult if I went blonde and I'd be back, 'having them done' in four weeks. As a former six monthly visitor to the salon, did I really wish to commit to the time and expense of that? She's a great hairdresser but I'm not sure she'll be vying for sales woman of the year any time soon.

So, what did I do? I went as dark as I could. And I almost quite like it.

And the other promises? I've been better with my zzzzs, my prosecco units have been low – most of the time – and *most* evenings I switch my phone off at 9pm. Honest.

Can you forgive me for forgoing the bleach?

It does grow back

Allow yourself to lament the passing of your hair, use painkillers if your scalp hurts, and scowl in the mirror if your reflection doesn't fill you with delight – but remember, your hair does grow back and with it you have the chance for a new style and colour, not to mention a condition and shine which your hair last saw when you were a baby.

The first tufts of my new hair started to sprout three weeks after the end of radiotherapy. We were off! Normal life was returning, or perhaps post breast cancer life was starting. And at a pace. Incidentally, I've learnt that my re-growth two months after the end of chemo was quite late. Lots of people

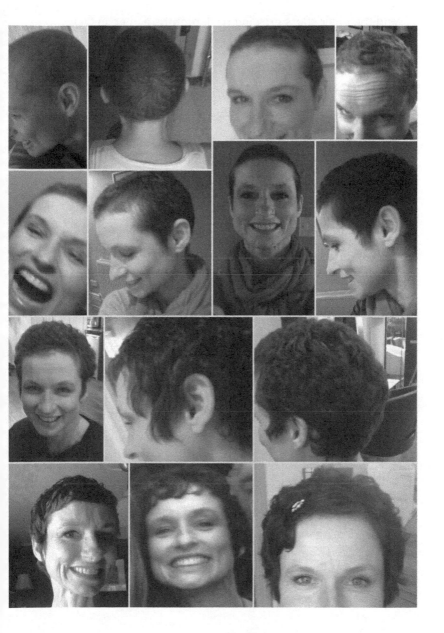

Fighting Cancer, Living Life

find their hair starts growing back months earlier, in fact, during their last few sessions of chemo. I had a few glimpses of hair during chemo, too, but it would promptly full out again after the next dose.

And if you're thinking my hair doesn't look too long for eight months of growth, don't despair, I've had it cut four times already. I didn't feel ready to cope with the 'growing out' stage straightaway. Having had over a year of no, or little, hair, I thought I'd give myself a breather before embarking on the unkempt passage to my shoulders and looking like the woman who time forgot. But now I'm impatient and as my hairdresser says, I have 'difficult hair to wear short'. What she means is that like my eyebrows, it grows sideways rather than downwards.

So, my short hair is now officially being, 'grown out'. Please be kind to me if you see me sporting a microphone head. I'm not relishing this stage. But I'm happy that I have got to a point in my cancer treatment where the state of my hair is of such importance.

Ditching the wig

Something I hadn't considered when I first wore my wig in public (feeling incredibly self-conscious, even though clearly no strangers could tell, and the people I knew all seemed to like the new and different me) was that one day I've be nervous about NOT wearing the wig anymore

Sometime in late August when I had my proud new tufts of hair over which my wig was still sitting at all times in public, I had my perfect opportunity to reveal the scant hair look. An invitation to my friend's 40th birthday party arrived, fancy dress, 80s style. Typical, I said to my teenage children, I've sported a stuck-in-The-Eighties-time-warp-mop my whole life that cries out for an Eighties Party, and when it comes, I haven't got 'the hair' anymore. Well, I said, I could always go as Sinead O'Connor.

Oh!

Of course we had to google Sinead O'Connor for their benefit but as we flicked through a photo montage, I couldn't help wondering if my flip comment might not be so ridiculous after all. I hadn't noticed back in the 80s that she was small, as I am (5 foot 1 to be precise), and that she had green eyes, as I do, not to mention a pale complexion like me. I even wondered if my face was a similar shape but kept that to myself as I felt faintly ridiculous comparing my 45 year old bald, tearful, eyelash and eyebrow-less face with that of the beautiful 20-something year old, Sinead O'Connor. Then came the crunch. If you do that Mum, I will be so impressed, said my eldest. So now I had no choice. I had to do it, but on one proviso – I had to have a complete covering of hair by party time. I didn't want anyone feeling sorry for me.

As the party drew closer and my costume sorted itself with great ease – black polo neck jumper, black jeans and purple DM boots, the latter being a much coveted loan from a friend who, alas, wasn't prepared to give them up on a permanent basis – I was really coming around to the idea. I'd enjoyed wearing my wigs but after six months, I was bored of them. The idea of sourcing an 80s style wig to wear to the party certainly didn't hold the excitement or amusement it would have done a year ago. Meanwhile, I had the prerequisite covering of hair and felt that for the first time in my fancy dress history, I had a costume I wouldn't need to explain to kind but puzzled party-goers.

When I arrived at the party with my bald-ish head on view for a hundred people to witness, I suddenly felt very, very bare. Even when I saw some ugly Margaret Thatchers with their hooked, wart covered noses, gooey foundation and American Tan tights, not to mention Vyvyan of The Young Ones – terrifically authentic but no oil painting – I still wondered if I had time to run home and change. I didn't run home, but only for fear of being rude.

So, here's the thing. When you out your new look in front of friends, it's a captive audience. Everybody can imagine how difficult it would be to lose their hair in such dramatic fashion, particularly, but not exclusively, as a woman. Our hair is a reflection of our personality. Never have I been more sure of this since losing mine. And people don't like others to feel sad or awkward, and will make a great effort to make you feel otherwise. The party was wonderful. I felt liberated to be dancing without my wig and went to bed with cheek bone ache from laughing.

Meanwhile my husband got to wear my day wig to complete his Bjorn Borg outfit. I couldn't possibly say whether his outfit was the best of the night, but I'd bet on his wig being the most expensive.

4. Positive Stories

When I was diagnosed with cancer, I wanted to hear success stories. I didn't know where to look for them and my efforts tended to turn up people who were struggling. Since then I've found a whole heap of them and I thought I'd share some with you. Not all the stories are about primary breast cancer but they are all about people out-living cancer. The following are real stories from real people:

Ali:

My mum had a brain tumour in her 30's and was a lucky one. She was diagnosed in 1985 aged 33. Thankfully her tumour was benign but a major op and months of radiotherapy followed. Much to my amusement (aged 11) she had a wonderful 1980s wig, a massive scar capable of scaring small children and hair that grew back a completely different colour. 30 years later, she's still here, fully appreciates that she was a lucky one and enjoys the simple pleasures of life. She tells me a smile from one of her grandchildren is enough to make her day!

Nicola:

My mum was 49 when diagnosed with a lump, 'the size of an orange' and lymph node involvement. She's just celebrated her 70th birthday.

Silvie:

My mum had breast cancer in 2001 and no recurrence. It's very unlikely to recur after so long.

Melissa:

I met the youngest looking 78 year old uni-boober today. It has been seven or eight years since her mastectomy, prior to that she had a lumpectomy with chemo and radiotherapy 4 years earlier. She says she feels fit, flat and fabulous thanks to healthy eating and gentle exercise.

Lucy:

My aunty had breast cancer nearly twenty years ago and is now in her 70's and fit as a fiddle. And my cousin also had cancer. They found it just after she had her second baby and she had to have chemo. A few years later she fell pregnant naturally and her third child is nearly twenty.

Paula:

My Nana, Sarah Violet Grey (or Violet), was diagnosed and treated for cancer of the leg in the 1960s. She had her calf removed and radiotherapy and lived a full and active life until 1992 when she died of natural causes, aged 79.

Amanda:

My mum, Doris, was diagnosed with breast cancer in 1990 and had a full mastectomy. She was re-diagnosed in 2013 with terminal secondary breast cancer and given only a short time to live. She's still showing no signs of even being ill at all! Still golfing, still loving and living life to the full and still has the mantra that the big C won't beat her. Even through her adversity, she continues to be my strength, my rock and my inspiration.

Treacy:

A good friend of mine, Liz, was diagnosed with a very aggressive tumour back in 2007 – she was only in her early 30's. A mastectomy was followed by chemo, but it has never slowed her down, and she travels all over the country working in security. This week she has finally been given the all-clear!

Deborah:

Boom. Easter 2012. 'I am very sorry, the cells we examined are not normal. They are cancer'. I was 42 years old with a 2 year and 5 year old. Fast forward 18 months. My aunt, cousin and I are all at the breast clinic. We joke that we should have a family bench. The bad news is that we do cancer really well in my family. Ovarian or breast cancer has taken a few of us – my dear mother in October last year and her mother the year before. The good news is that we are forewarned and forearmed now. My aunt is doing well (though she is not genetically significant to me, she is a hugely significant person in my life). She has no evidence of disease after 10 years and had bilateral breast cancer. My cousin's was found early following a routine mammogram. She too is doing well with a good prognosis. I am two years post diagnosis and have no evidence of disease. My younger sister gets annual mammograms now. We are all living life and hopeful that we have broken the cycle.

Yvonne:

My friend's mum had a double mastectomy when she was 43 and has just celebrated her 75th birthday and my cousin's friend was 38 when she was diagnosed and we just celebrated her 60th birthday. Both still going strong!

Dave:

My mum had lung cancer aged 79. She had an operation and to be on the safe side the surgeon took away half of her left lung. She was in intensive care for two days and in hospital for a week. No chemo or radiotherapy though. She refused to give in, has never moaned and appreciates she is perhaps one of the lucky ones. She is 83 now. I think this is a nice story for older people who get cancer later in life. Worth noting that the surgeon said he was prepared to operate only because he thought she had a chance of surviving the op – because he knew she had kept herself fit and healthy in later life. There's a message to people to look after themselves.

Jane:

My Auntie June had a double mastectomy in 1965 aged 30 and lived until she was 78.

Hannah:

*My husband's aunt was diagnosed at 45 and then again at 72...
she's still going strong at 85! She lives on her own and is such a
positive woman. Her secret? 'I just won't give in!'*

Antonia:

*My cousin, Margaret, from Nottinghamshire was diagnosed with
breast cancer 49 years ago. She had a double mastectomy. She is
now 78 and plays bridge, does flower arranging and organises me.
Awesome woman.*

Simonne:

*My Nan was diagnosed at 59 and had a lumpectomy and
radiotherapy. She is alive and kicking at 83.*

Lorraine:

My other half's gran had it 25 years ago and is now 85!

Positive Stories

5. Proceeds from Tea & Chemo

breast cancer now

Due to being diagnosed with breast cancer at the relatively young age of 45, I screeched into eligibility for the Young Breast Cancer Network (YBCN) before the 45 year old cut off. This private group on Facebook, now with thousands of members, was set up by Vicky Yates as a fun but supportive place to hang out for younger women diagnosed with breast cancer. Vicky was just 36 when she was diagnosed and found it difficult always being the youngest person at clinics. The group is a safe haven for young women finding themselves in the same position as Vicky was.

Through the site I have met some truly strong, positive and fun people, both on- and offline. However, this sanctuary has also opened me up to a world of sadness. Young women, really young women, who are a decade, sometimes almost a generation, younger than me, are diagnosed with breast cancer, only to hear what everybody fears, that their cancer has metastasized; they have secondaries. Many of these women are continuing to live for years after diagnosis which is inspiring in itself, but some of them have passed away.

Enormous progress has been made in the diagnosis, treatment and survival of people with cancer. It's a realistic hope that the day is coming when we might take a pill to blast every single speck of a cancer cell into cancer hell so that a diagnosis of cancer is never a death sentence any more. But we're not there yet.

A wonderful new charity was set up earlier in 2015 called Breast Cancer Now. It's an amalgamation of the two charities: Breast Cancer Campaign and Breakthrough Breast Cancer. Its aim is to consign deaths from secondary breast cancer to history by 2050. A powerful advert was designed featuring some people I've met in YBCN, together with other young women living with secondary breast cancer, which you can see here: **http://breastcancernow.org/**. It blew my mind. These women were saying that they wouldn't be the last people to die from breast cancer because the disease is too advanced in them. But somebody could be.

Some of my on-line friends from the group went to the launch of Breast Cancer Now and a great blogger, Diane Riley-Waite, posted eloquently here – **https://alittleearthquake.wordpress.com/2015/06/15/breast-cancer-now/**

I was inspired to help and this is why a third of the proceeds from *Tea & Chemo* will go to Breast Cancer Now. Wouldn't it be wonderful if our generation could change the course of the future? We have to try, don't we?

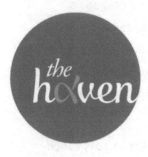

The Haven

I was diagnosed with breast cancer a few months after breaking my foot. I'd just started running again but after calling my husband to pick me up from where I was stranded with a foot which couldn't bear to touch the ground, I thought I'd better get back to physio. I'd had a few sessions and felt I was on the mend when my foot paled into comic insignificance following the, 'It's very aggressive, grade three, much worse than we thought', meeting.

I didn't know if a cancer diagnosis had any bearing on physio but as far as I was concerned, I was waiting for my mastectomy, hadn't started chemo, wasn't teaching and wanted to run. I also knew that if I could run during treatment, that it would help get me through. And it did.

So I kept my appointment with Helen, my physio.

Good Christmas? she asked.

A bit different, I said.

After years of chatter while Helen had pummelled my sore hamstrings, calf, other calf, bum and, oh, the pain, my back, she'd never told me about her auntie. Until now. I learnt she'd had breast cancer in her 50's and The Haven had been her auntie's, well, haven. Helen said that it had also been good for her as a relative. She said that I would have to go. I'd get lots of free treatments which would really help in chemo and I'd meet other people in the same situation. Right, I said. I didn't want to be rude but I intended on running my way through treatments and going for cappuccinos with my existing friends in between. I wasn't sure I'd have time to meet new people – or whether it would be helpful.

And you'll have to model in the annual fashion show, she said.

You can probably imagine how I felt about that. Aside from the fact that nothing ever fits me, walking down the stage with only one boob and a bald head? Thanks for the offer but I think I'll be at home pairing socks that night.

Back to the task in hand and the physical pummelling of strategic points in my legs. I was told that I wouldn't be able to have my usual physio that week but that Helen could gently massage the affected area in my foot, which sounded a fairly pleasant alternative.

The only hint Helen gave that my news had shocked her was when I became aware of her massaging the wrong foot. At first I wondered if this alternative to the tirade upon my hamstrings was a 2 for 1 deal, but when she tapped my foot and said, 'All done!' I realised that my fiercely organised physio was flustered.

Flash forward a year and yes, I did visit The Haven. On my first trip I sat for an hour with the manager, Debra Horsman, and cried. I didn't even think I was feeling upset and I very rarely cried about cancer in the early days. I was sent away with a programme of treatments including reflexology, acupuncture and a nutritional consultation. Nine months after diagnosis I was involved in my first ever fashion shoot, wig still firmly in place, for LK Bennett in aid of the Haven. And just over a year later I was part of the Bo Carter modelling group in the annual Haven Fashion Show, without the wig this time. It was the most uplifting experience and one I intend to repeat every year until they won't have me anymore. I hasten to add that the rigorous selection process for the modelling involved sending an RSVP to say I was available.

My physio was right. The Haven is a godsend for people with a cancer diagnosis and their family and friends. But it's totally reliant on fundraising.

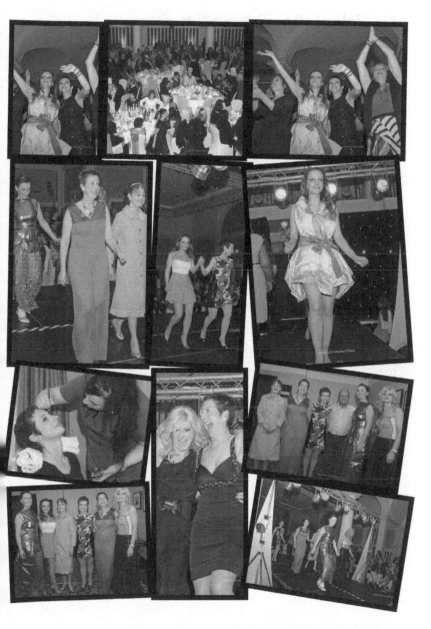

Proceeds from Tea & Chemo

Sir Robert Ogden Macmillan Centre in Harrogate

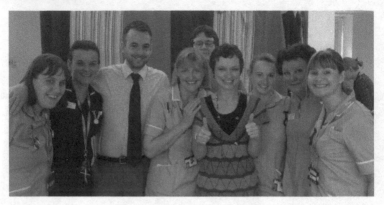

Because breast cancer is the most common cancer in women, and the second most common cause of cancer death in women (after lung cancer) in the UK, it isn't surprising it gains a lot of coverage and support. I have written primarily about breast cancer here because it is the cancer I understand most about. It would be wrong to try to second guess the side-effects and difficulties peculiar to people facing bowel cancer, for example, even though The Fear and the impact on our lives and on our friends and family will be similar.

A third of the proceeds of *Tea & Chemo* will go to the Sir Robert Ogden Macmillan Centre in Harrogate, which serves people with all types of cancer in this area of Yorkshire. The team of staff at the centre were responsible for turning the emotionally and physically difficult experience of having chemo into something almost pleasant – honestly. I never felt as secure and cared for as when I was attending the Centre every three weeks. Indeed, when I was pronounced unsuitable for the injection of Herceptin to be administered at home, and instead would need to continue attending the hospital every three weeks for a year to receive it intravenously, nobody was more pleased than me. I'd like some of the proceeds of *Tea & Chemo* to go to the department to show my gratitude to all the staff and volunteers, and also as an attempt to do something small for all cancer sufferers and their loved ones.

6. A Final Word

People ask me if I ever get down about cancer, adding that they're sure I must do sometimes. I'm glad that the general impression seems to be that I don't, but I do get myself in a bit of a grump now and again. More often, however, I get cross. I get cross that cancer exists. I get cross that it still kills people. And I get cross about the impact cancer has had on my life, and that of my husband and children, both during and post active treatment; and the effect it will continue to have in years to come. I also don't care much for the gloominess which The Fear can sometimes cast.

I don't feel cross or sad in a, 'why me?' kind of way though. Cancer exists, like dementia and heart disease, cartilage tears and colds, Parkinson's and motor neurone disease. How can I feel sorry for myself when I look at what Stephen Hawking has done with his life, despite contracting his disease at 21? And there are many far lower profile people living with motor neurone disease every day and they will have their life dramatically cut short by it.

I once worked with a man in his 20's and he had severe cerebral palsy, referring to it as 'CP' (which made it sound less serious somehow). He volunteered for a charity where I worked in PR and fundraising and turned my scribblings and photos into beautiful reports and brochures. I was totally in awe of this man. He rarely spoke about his disability even though it clearly impacted on his every day; eating, drinking, moving, speaking. In a rare chat about living with his disabilities, and when he was talking about what CP enabled him to do – not, I noted, what CP prevented him doing – he said, You're going to ask me whether I'd prefer to be able-bodied or have CP aren't you? I smiled to myself, clocked my ignorant assumptions. No, I wasn't going to ask that. Nobody would choose having disabilities over being able-bodied, would they? Being able-bodied was just so much, well, easier.

CP, he said. No one believes me but I'd prefer to have CP than be able-bodied.

It's rare for me to be stuck for a response but I was. To be able to see life in this way, to have so much positive thinking, was stunning. If you wanted to argue it logically you could say that he couldn't possibly comment because he hadn't known life without CP, but I think this is irrelevant. The point is that his perception of his life was positive and that was his reality. This was what he truly believed and it made him happy. True happiness really is a matter of perception.

I wrote a blog post on, 'true happiness' before cancer was even a suspicion in my life. I used to say that you had to be 'down to be up'. I still believe that. How do you recognise true happiness if you don't have a little glimmer of more difficult times for comparison? If I was on a cloud looking down, I'd probably miss the disgruntled moments, angry outbursts, sad times even, because they are living, aren't they? They are part of it. I remember my lovely octogenarian neighbour talking of her sadness years after the death of her husband, and she said that she even missed arguing with him. And I understand that. Why don't we want to die? Because we like living, warts and all.

In recent years I've learned a better phrase for the less memorable, 'down to be up': Life isn't about waiting for the storm to pass it's about learning to dance in the rain.

I worry that we are teaching a generation of children that life always has to be 'good', otherwise it's failing us and we should feel badly done by. But 'good' is only a matter of perception. Good is the whole picture, not simply a part. It's recognising closeness and support in difficult times. It's treasuring the love and support of friends and family when we're feeling rough. It's recognising that we can still walk, speak, function, laugh when we lose our job and who knows, it might lead to something even better. I don't believe true happiness lies in anything tangible, nice though holidays and a comfortable home are, but in our perception of our environment and the people who dance with us in it. I have a great house and have no desire to move – ever. But it isn't the walls, it's the people within and around them and the conversation, laughs (and arguments) we have which make me glad to be alive.

I think happiness is quite straightforward really. I think it lies in seeing the glass half full and instinctively looking for the silver lining. Do this, and in my humble opinion you can get through anything. Having cancer has made me believe this even more fervently than I did before.

After all, you get a cup of tea with chemo.

7. Appendix

This is not an exhaustive list of terms and organisations involved with cancer, but an appendix of terms used in *Tea & Chemo*. The large charities mentioned will all provide more in-depth information and links to their websites are included here.

Alcohol – to better understand units and for more information on safe drinking, visit:

http://www.drinkaware.co.uk/

Blood Donor – blood donors are always needed. See: **www.blood.co.uk**

Bone Marrow Donor – the more people on the register, the more lives saved. See: **www.anthonynolan.org**

Breast Cancer Care – striving to achieve the best treatment, information and support for every person affected by breast cancer. My go-to place for a sense-check on facts and figures: **https://www.breastcancercare.org.uk**

Breast Cancer Now – formed in 2015 from an amalgamation of the two charities, Breast Cancer Campaign and Breakthrough Breast Cancer. Its goal is to see an end to all deaths from secondary breast cancer by 2015. Visit: **http://breastcancernow.org**

Breast Cancer Nurse (BCN) – a key worker assigned to you. She/he will be your first port of call throughout your cancer treatment.

Breast Cancer UK – for information on perceived carcinogens and hazardous chemicals: **http://www.breastcanceruk.org.uk**

Cancer Research UK – the world's leading charity dedicated to beating cancer through research. Another sane but sympathetic site where stats are well hidden: **www.cancerresearchuk.org**

Cancerversary – a term coined to celebrate a year since a cancer diagnosis.

Chillow Pillow – a cold pillow useful in preventing or decreasing the number of 'warm flushes' at night. See Warm Flush in *A Little Less Squished*.

Haven (the) – a 'haven' offering additional support to those affected by breast cancer. Visit: **www.thehaven.org.uk**

Flat Friends – an on-line group for people who have decided against reconstruction. Visit: **http://www.flatfriends.org.uk**

Herceptin (Trastuzumab) – a treatment given in the case of HER2 positive breast cancers (where breast cancer cells have more HER2 receptors which can make the cancer cells grow more quickly.)

Holistic Treatments – a form of healing which considers the whole person; body, mind and spirit. See: Mindfulness, Acupuncture and Reflexology in The New Normal.

Lumpectomy – an operation in which only part of the breast is removed.

Lymphoedema – a dibilitating pooling of the lymph fluid. A post-operative risk. See *Blood, Blood, Glorious Blood.*

Macmillan Cancer Support – helping patients and their loved ones face cancer from diagnosis to treatment and beyond. Visit: **http://www.macmillan.org.uk**

Marie Curie Cancer Care – helping people living with terminal illness and their families.
Visit: **www.mariecurie.org.uk**

Mastectomy – an operation in which the entire breast is removed. See The not knowing in *Pebbles* and To reconstruct or not to reconstruct in *Why Not Me?*

Multidisciplinary Team (MDT) – a group of specialists in different areas of cancer treatment and care who meet to discuss best practice.

Menopause – see The new normal *in A Little Less Squished.*

NHS Choices – a one-stop site for sensible information on all areas of health. Visit: **http://www.nhs.uk**

Oncologist – a member of staff assigned to the treatment side of your cancer care.

Parabens – additives to help prolong the life of toiletries. See *Your Personality in Your Hands*.

Pathology Report – a statement on the size, type and stage of your cancer. See The not knowing in *Pebbles*.

Premature menopause – see The new normal *in A Little Less Squished*.

Race for Life – organised by Cancer Research UK who receive no government funding. See *Tutus Ready? And We're Off!* **http://raceforlife.cancerresearchuk.org/**

Reconstruction – see *Why Not Me?*

Reflexology – see The new normal *in A Little Less Squished*.

Scarves – see *Your Personality in your Hands* for useful links.

Sir Robert Ogden Macmillan Centre – Harrogate Hospital's centre for cancer treatment. See *Proceeds from Tea & Chemo*. **http://www.hdft.nhs.uk/**

Tamoxifen – a form of hormone therapy used in oestrogen receptor-positive breast cancer. Tamoxifen blocks oestrogen from reaching the cancer cells which can reduce the speed of the growth of cancer cells or prevent it altogether.

Younger Breast Cancer Network (YBCN) – a private group on Facebook open to anybody diagnosed with breast cancer under the age of 45. This link takes you to its public page where you will then be able to register with the private group: **https://m.facebook.com/ YoungerBreastCancerNetwork**

Wigs – see *Your Personality in your Hands* and *Gone Dark Brown* for useful links and information.

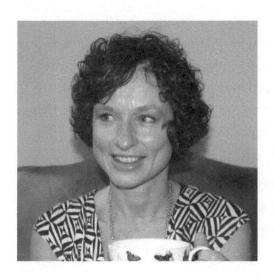

Jackie Buxton is a writer, editor and teacher of creative writing. She is currently working on her second novel and her first, Glass Houses, is to be published in 2016 by Urbane Publications. First chapters of both have won or been placed in the Retreat West, Oxford Editors' and Writers' Billboard competitions. Jackie's short stories feature in three anthologies, on-line and in Chase Magazine, for which she also writes a bi-monthly double page spread of book reviews.

Jackie's blog, *Agenthood and Submissionville*, evolved from a wry look at the world of novel submission for publication, into a pot pourri of stories of the strange things which happen while she's trying to write or bring up her children. Diagnosed with an aggressive form of breast cancer in December 2013,

Jackie decided to blog about her experience of living with cancer and its nine months of treatments. The result is a candid, often humorous, insight into a time she nicknames, Not All Bad. Motivated by reader enthusiasm to publish a book based on her blog, *Tea & Chemo: Fighting Cancer, Living Life* is a patchwork of positivity and resource for those living with cancer, as well as for their family and friends.

Jackie lives in Yorkshire with her husband and teenage children and when not writing, can often be found cycling, running, dreaming or tripping up through the beautiful Yorkshire Dales.

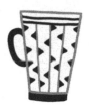

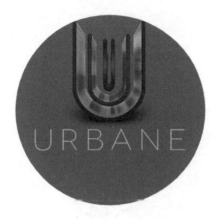

Urbane Publications is dedicated to
developing new author voices, and publishing
fiction and non-fiction that challenges, thrills and
fascinates.
From page-turning novels to innovative
reference books, our goal is to publish what
YOU want to read.

Find out more at
urbanepublications.com